A COLOR ATLAS OF BREAST HISTOPATHOLOGY

A COLOR ATLAS OF BREAST HISTOPATHOLOGY

M. Trojani
Laboratory of Pathological Anatomy
Bordeaux
France

J. B. LIPPINCOTT COMPANY *Philadelphia*

Original French language edition (Atlas en couleurs d'histopathologie mammaire)
© 1988 Éditions Maloine

English edition 1991

© 1991 Chapman and Hall

Distributed in the USA and Canada
by J. B. Lippincott Company,
East Washington Square,
Philadelphia, PA 19105, USA

Printed and bound in France

ISBN 0-397-58319-2

Library of Congress Catalog Card Number

90-60686

Contents

PREFACE

Dr Trojani heads the Pathology Unit at the Foundation Bergonié Cancer Center, Bordeaux, and has for several years been using demonstrative photographs of various mammary lesions in her teaching. In doing so, she has gathered a wide range of mammographic, macroscopic and histological images. The idea of making a whole atlas from this collection of pedagogic documents required completion by a set of comparable documents, covering normal structures, and dystrophic and neoplastic breast pathology.

A Colour Atlas of Breast Histopathology provides students, pathologists, oncologists, gynaecologists, senologists and other specialists with a reference tool and comprises a clear, concise commentary parallel to the figures and their captions. The text is fully up to date regarding nosologic notions and discusses differences of terminology existing in current practice. Particular modifications of current debate such as proliferative disease of the breast, lobular carcinoma *in situ* and ductal carcinoma *in situ* figure prominently, to the satisfaction, I'm sure, of all.

I am especially pleased to be able to congratulate Dr Trojani on having successfully completed such a demanding project; she has worked with competence, tenacity and rigor, particularly in the choice of her graphic material.

I wish this atlas of mammary pathology all the success it deserves; the great assistance it will provide will be felt in more than one medical field.

F. Cabanne

LIST OF ABBREVIATIONS

AB	alcian blue
ADH	atypical ductal hyperplasia
ALH	atypical lobular hyperplasia
AML	acute myeloid leukaemia
BDA	blunt duct adenosis
C	carcinoma
Cytok	cytokeratin
DCIS	ductal carcinoma in situ
D-PAS	diastase-PAS
EMA	epithelial membrane antigen
FCD	fibrocystic disease
GCDFP-15	gross cystic disease fluid protein-15
HE	hematoxylin-eosin
HES	hematoxylin-eosin-safran
ID	intraductal
IDC-NOS	invasive ductal carcinoma not otherwise specified
IDC-pred ID	invasive ductal carcinoma with a predominant intraductal component
ILC	invasive lobular carcinoma
LCA	leucocyte common antigen
LCIS	lobular carcinoma in situ
MGG	May-Grünwald-Giemsa
NHML	non-Hodgkin's malignant lymphoma
PAS	periodic acid-Schiff
TDLU	terminal ductal-lobular unit
Vim	vimentin
WHO	World Health Organization

INTRODUCTION

This atlas originated with a few slides used to illustrate some difficult breast lesions to students. In view of their positive response, I have completed the iconography over the years and added a brief text indicating for each lesion the synonyms, the nosological difficulties and the main clinical, radiological and histological characteristics. The classification of tumours published by the World Health Organization in 1981 served as a guide to the presentation of the atlas. The photographs are from slides (24 × 36) taken with a ZEISS photomicroscope on Kodachrome 25 film. For each photograph, the staining technique used and the magnification of the photomicroscope are indicated. In routine study, slides are stained by hematoxylin-eosin-safran. Other staining techniques used are periodic acid-Schiff, periodic acid-Schiff-diastasis, periodic acid-Schiff-alcian blue, Grimelius and Shikata orcein. Immunohistochemical stainings are performed with monoclonal antibodies (anti cytokeratin (KL1 Immunotech), anti-epithelial membrane antigen (Dako), anti-leucocyte common antigen (Dako), antivimentine (Dako), or polyclonal antibodies (anti-S100 protein (Dako)) according to a three-stage immunoperoxidase procedure using diaminobenzidine to stimulate the peroxidase activity. General references to publications of breast pathology are presented at the beginning of the atlas. References to articles related to subject matter are found at the end of each chapter.

Among the many colleagues and associated staff who helped to contribute to the preparation of the atlas, I wish to pay special thanks to the following individuals:

Professor F. Cabanne for his invaluable advice and support, without which this atlas would never have been published. Although I have never studied under him, his numerous papers have always aroused my strongest and respectful admiration;

Mr P. Guillaumat, president of the 'Ligue nationale française contre le cancer' and Mr J.F. Duplan, president of the 'Comité départemental de la Gironde, Ligue nationale française contre le cancer', whose grant enabled the publication of this atlas;

Professor C. Lagarde, Head of the 'Fondation Bergonié' until 1986, and Professor D. Marée, his successor, for providing the necessary working environment to undertake this work;

My colleagues I. De Mascarel and J.M. Coindre for their constant support.

Glossary

Clinical terms

Occult cancer: a non palpable cancer, at times not detectable by mammography.

Early cancer: cancer detected at an early stage. This term is mainly used clinically and is related to small tumours or for carcinomas of any size with non axillary or distant metastases. It is an incorrect term because it does not take account of the cell kinetic study of tumour growth. In histology, it is also used for the malignant features of breast lesions difficult to diagnose. There is controversy whether these features are an early stage of carcinoma or represent a particular appearance of it.

Inflammatory carcinoma (mastitis carcinomatosa): clinical form of cancer which presents with oedema and redness of the skin as well as tenderness and rapid enlargement of the breast. The prognosis is poor with early nodal and distant metastases. Survival is very short, despite any form of treatment. This carcinoma is most often associated with dermal lymphatic invasion.

'Primary radiation therapy': combination of conservative surgery, i.e. resection of the primary tumour, and radiation therapy for the eradication of residual, multifocal and/or multicentric foci in the breast and sometimes in the nodal areas.

Histological terms

In situ carcinoma or preinvasive carcinoma: intraductal or lobular proliferation without visible invasion, when viewed by light microscopy.

Microinvasive intraductal carcinoma: see Chapter 7, page 168.

Minimal breast cancer: includes non-invasive carcinoma, either ductal or lobular, and invasive carcinoma measuring less than 10mm in diameter. Some authors include low-grade carcinomas such as adenoid cystic, mucinous, medullary or tubular forms.

Local invasion of the breast tumour (or spread of the tumour within the breast):
- *multicentric:* evaluated on a sufficient number of sections; corresponds to the presence of carcinoma of the same histological type within a quadrant other than that of the tumour or within the nipple (central tumours or nipple involvement by contiguity excluded). Some authors prefer a definition based on the distance between two carcinomatous foci (>5cm) or on the presence of normal breast tissue between the foci.
- *multifocal:* distinct carcinomatous foci localized near or in the same quadrant as the main tumour (Fisher, 1986).
- *residual foci:* carcinomatous foci near the original tumour site following excision.

Lobular cancer: see Chapter 7, page 138.

Pagetoid spread: this term indicates the presence of foreign cells within duct epithelium, similar to Paget cells in the epidermis. Pagetoid spread appears as one or several cell layers localized beneath the inner epithelial layer. Proliferation remains intraepithelial for a long time, then gradually displaces the epithelium, destroys it and fills up the lumen.

Occult invasion: ductal carcinoma in situ; two possible interpretations:
- an inverse process not visible by light microscopy and diagnosed by nodal metastases, or
- an invasive focus found in the mastectomy specimen while the excised tumour was only a ductal carcinoma in situ.

Axillary nodal metastasis: defined by metastasis diameter (Huvos, 1970) applicable for routine studies of a median section of lymph node stained by hematoxylin-eosin-safran:

- macrometastasis >2mm
- micrometastasis <2mm
- occult micrometastasis: not detected by routine examination; a metastasis detected by serial sections has a size from 0.22 to 1.3mm in Fisher's series (1978). It can now be detected by immunohistochemical staining using monoclonal antibodies against epithelial antigens. They are very small because they are composed of single cells or a few clusters of cells.

Surgical terms

Numerous and often vague for describing the actual excision.

Radical mastectomy: total mastectomy with axillary dissection. Two types of radical mastectomy:
- Halsted type: aggressive local operation removing simultaneously breast, pectoralis muscles and axillary lymph nodes. This operation was based on the concept that the breast carcinoma was a locoregional disease, thus requiring a large excision. It has now largely been abandoned.
- modified type: also known as total mastectomy with axillary dissection, removing separately breast (without pectoralis muscles) and axillary lymph nodes. It is now the standard procedure for mastectomy. Axillary dissection is performed not only for control of local disease (as Halsted did), but for establishing prognosis and the use of adjuvant therapy.

Limited surgery: many terms are used which mean excision of the tumour and breast tissue in varying amounts depending on the tumour and breast sizes: lumpectomy, segmental mastectomy, tylectomy, quadrantectomy, tumourectomy, partial mastectomy. In the breast carcinoma, this conservative surgery is generally associated with axillary dissection and adjuvant therapy. It is based on the concept of a systemic disease with possible distant metastases at the time of surgery. In this case, major surgery would not result in a greater likelihood of recovery than limited surgery.

General references

Ahmed, A. Atlas of the ultrastructure of human breast diseases. New York, Churchill Livingstone, 1978.

Azzopardi, J.G. Problems in breast pathology, Philadelphia, W.B. Saunders, 1979.

Cabanne, F., Bonenfant, J.-L. Anatomie pathologique. Québec, Presses de l'Université, Laval et Paris, Maloine, 1982, 2ᵉ édition, pp. 1213–1231.

Fisher, E.R., Gregorio, R.M., Fisher, B. The pathology of invasive breast cancer. A syllabus derived from findings of the National Surgical Adjuvant Breast Project (protocol nᵒ 4) *Cancer*, 1975, **36**, 1–85.

Foote, F.W., Stewart, F.W. Comparative studies of cancerous versus non cancerous breasts. I. Basic morphologic characteristics. *Ann. Surg.*, 1945, **121**, 6–53.

II. Role of so-called chronic cystic mastitis in mammary carcinogenesis. Influence of certain hormones on human breast structure. *Ann. Surg.*, 1945, **121**, 197–222.

Haagensen, C.D. Diseases of the breast. Third Edition. Philadelphia. W.B. Saunders, 1986.

Haagensen, C.D., Bodian, C., Haagensen, D.E. Breast carcinoma. Risk and detection. Philadelphia. W.B. Saunders, 1981.

Linell, F., Ljungberg, O., Andersson, I. Breast carcinoma. Aspects of early stages, progression and related problems. *Acta Pathol. Microbiol. Scand.* (A), 1980, suppl. 272.

McDivitt, R.W., Stewart, F.W., Berg, J.W. Tumors of the breast. Atlas of tumor pathology, second series, fasc. 2, Washington D.C., Armed Forces Institute of Pathology, 1968.

Scarff, W., Torloni, H. Types histologiques des tumeurs du sein. Classification histologique internationale des tumeurs; nᵒ 2, Genève, O.M.S., 1981, 2ᵉ édition.

Wellings, S.R., Jensen, H.M., Marcum, R.G. An atlas of subgross pathology of the human breast with special reference to possible precancerous lesions. *J. Nat. Cancer Inst.*, 1975, **55**, 231–273.

1

Normal breast

1.1 NOMENCLATURE OF THE MAIN ANATOMICAL PART OF THE BREAST. CORRELATIONS WITH HISTOLOGY

The terminology varies considerably depending on the authors and each term has to be clearly defined.

Duct segmentation
Nine to ten ducts (termed major, large, collecting, segmental, or subareolar) open to the nipple by a separate orifice. They include a dilated part with sinuous contours termed lactiferous or milk sinus. Then they divide into medium (or subsegmental) and small ducts ending in:

The terminal ductal-lobular unit (TDLU) (Wellings, 1975) which contains the extra and intralobular terminal ducts ending in the smallest epithelial structure within the lobule: the terminal ductule or acinus. Acini are probably functional only during pregnancy and lactation.

1 Diagram of duct segmentation.

2 Diagram of the TDLU.

3 HES ×10
Lactiferous or milk sinus (not to be mistaken for a papillomatous hyperplasia).

4 HES ×64
Large duct with two cell layers, an epithelial inner and a myoepithelial outer layer.

5 HES ×64
6 Orcein ×64
Large duct: periductal elastosis increasing with age and parity.

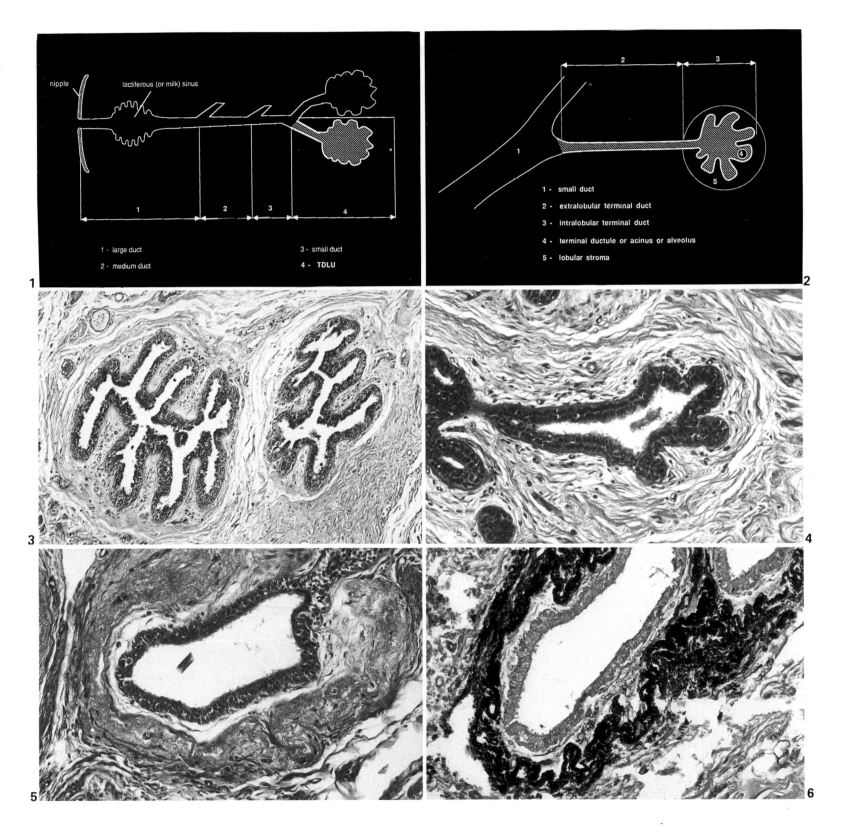

1 - large duct
2 - medium duct
3 - small duct
4 - TDLU

1 - small duct
2 - extralobular terminal duct
3 - intralobular terminal duct
4 - terminal ductule or acinus or alveolus
5 - lobular stroma

7 HES ×64
Small duct with myoid differentiation of the myo-epithelial cell layer.

8 S100 Protein ×64
Positive myoepithelial cells in a small duct.

9 HES ×25
TDLU (terminal ductal-lobular unit).

10 Orcein ×25
Elastic tissue surrounds the extralobular terminal duct but is absent within the lobule.

11 HES ×160
Myoid differentiation of myoepithelial cells with particular eosinophilic globules.

12 S100 Protein ×160
Positive myoepithelial cells in the acini.

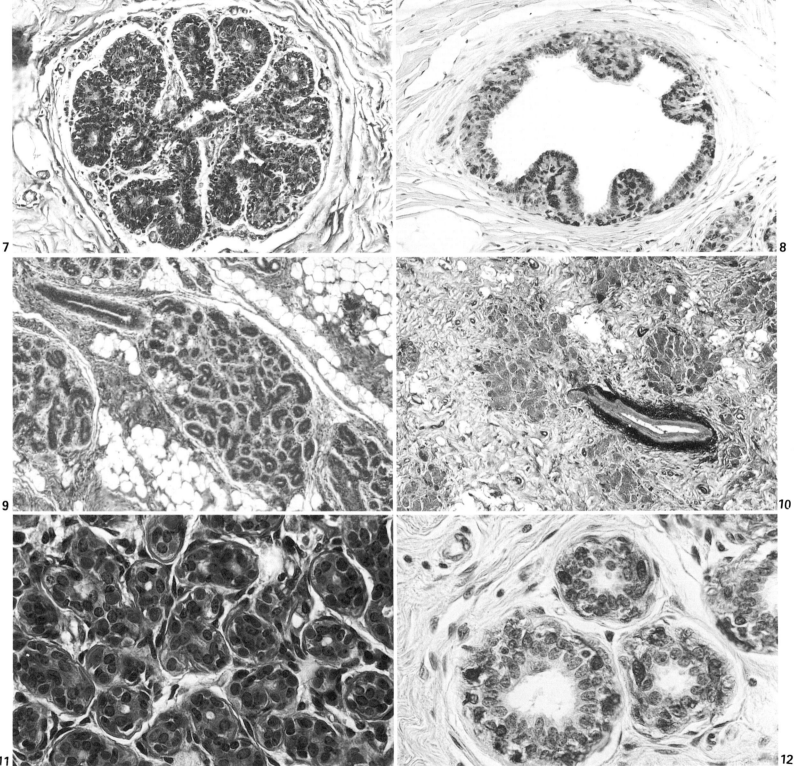

1.2 SOME PHYSIOLOGICAL ASPECTS OF BREAST TISSUE

13 HES ×25
Normal breast tissue with regular size and distribution of lobules.

14 HES ×25
Atrophic breast tissue.

15 HES ×64
16 HES ×160
Involutive lobule: small acini are surrounded by a thick sclerohyaline layer.

17 HES ×25
18 HES ×160
A secretory lobule: acini are dilated and the epithelial cells have a vacuolated cytoplasm. This lobular change may be:
- diffuse in the breast during pregnancy and lactation;
- focal, either by a selective susceptibility of individual lobules to endogenous hormones, or by exogenous hormonal treatment (these changes have been observed in men during oestrogen therapy for prostatic cancer).

References
Chap. 1 – Normal breast

Longgacre, P.A. *et al.* (1986) A correlative morphologic study of human breast and endometrium in the menstrual cycle. *Am. J. Surg. Pathol.*, **10**, 382.

Tavassoli, F.A. *et al.* (1987) Lactational and clear cell changes of the breast in non lactating, non pregnant women. *Am. J. Clin. Pathol.*, **87**, 23.

Van Bogaert, L.J. (1984) Glande mammaire: développement embryonnaire et foetal, anatomie, micro-anatomie. *Rev. Fr. Gynécol., Obstet.*, **79**, 159.

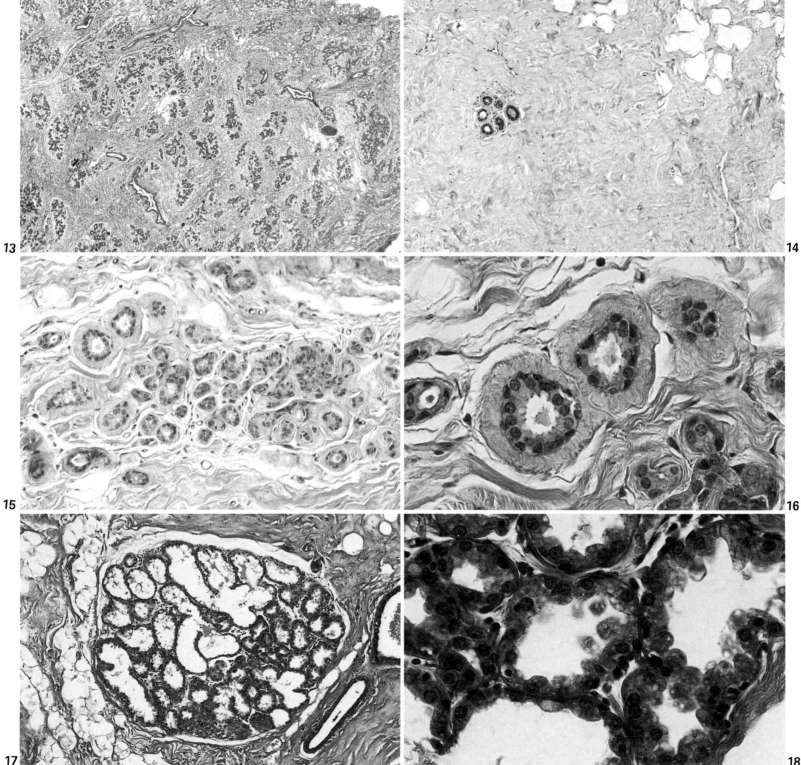

2

Fibrocystic disease

Synonyms

'Mazoplasia', chronic mastitis, dysplasia, fibroadenosis, mastopathy.

Definition

Benign lesion including cyst, fibrosis, lobular or ductal epithelial hyperplasia. One of these components may be predominant.

This traditional definition is currently disputed because the term of fibrocystic disease includes a lot of different lesions, only a few of which constitute risk factors for breast cancer. Some authors wish this term to be suppressed and replaced by a specific histologic designation based on the proliferative activity of mammary epithelium.

'Let's say good-bye to fibrocystic disease, truly a non-disease, and begin to deal with proliferative disease of the breast' (Hutter, 1985).

However, the disorders usually classed in fibrocystic disease (FCD) will be studied in this chapter. Proliferative atypical lesions, i.e. atypical ductal or lobular hyperplasia, will be studied with corresponding carcinomas in situ.

2.1   Cyst
2.2   Epitheliosis (papillomatosis)
2.3   Adenosis
2.4   Radial scar

2.1 CYST

Cysts are classified according to size as microcysts if smaller than 3mm in diameter and gross cysts if 3mm or more in diameter.

Origin

From lobules or small ducts which end blindly in blunt duct adenosis. For Wellings (1984) (see diagram below), cysts are the endpoint of progressive 'unfolding' of lobules due to the accumulation of secretions (epithelial hyperplasia or fibrous obliteration of the lumina of small ducts may prevent fluid reabsorption).

Progressive unfolding of lobule:
cyst formation (*Wellings*)

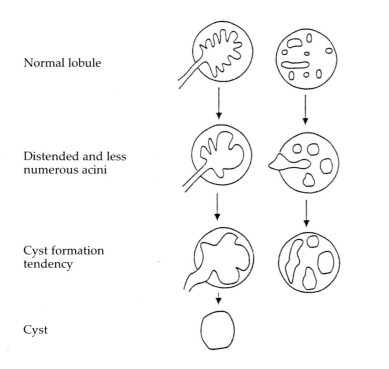

Normal lobule

Distended and less numerous acini

Cyst formation tendency

Cyst

Microcysts are not palpable and are so frequent that they do not probably represent a real breast disease. They are lined by non-apocrine or apocrine, flattened or papillary epithelium.

19 Typical bluish colour of a cyst as revealed at operation.

20 HES ×25
Microcyst with non-apocrine epithelium.

21 HES ×25
Microcysts with apocrine epithelium.

22 HES ×25
Microcysts with proliferative papillary apocrine metaplasia.

23 HES ×160
Apocrine cells contain granules close to the luminal margins and have round nuclei with prominent nucleoli.

24 D-PAS ×160
PAS-positive diastase-resistant granules close to the luminal margins.

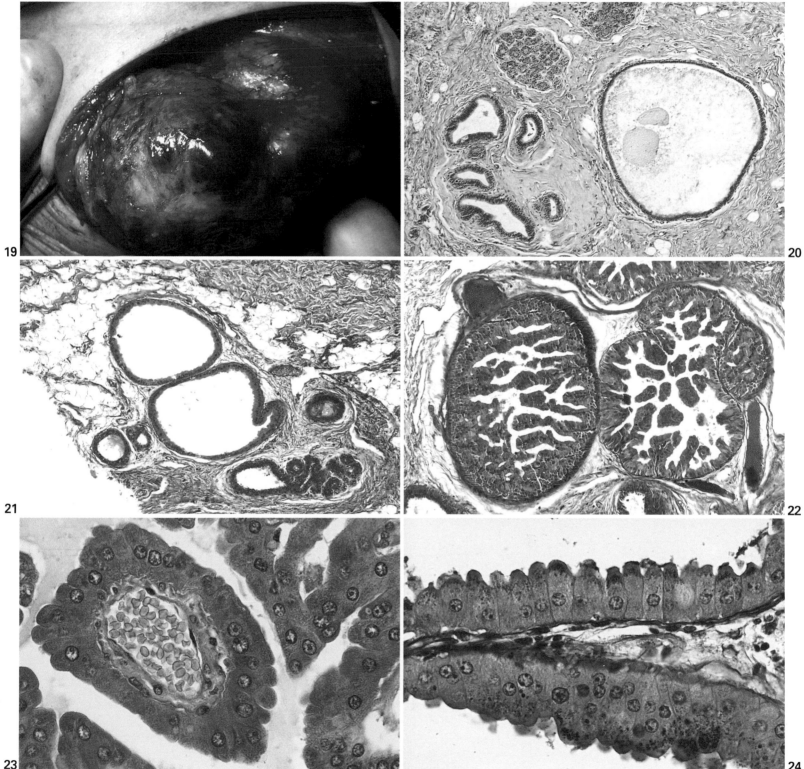

Gross cysts are usually palpable and occur in the breast of about 7% of women. They vary in size, enlarging rapidly in the premenstrual phase and becoming painful (due to the tension of the fluid within the cyst). But they may decrease in size and even disappear.

Pathology

- Tension cysts: the apocrine epithelium is detached from the wall which has only a lining of compressed fibrous tissue with or without an inflammatory infiltrate. The fluid of a tension cyst contains a protein (GCDFP-15) which appears as an apocrine marker.
- Ruptured tension cysts: the apocrine epithelium is destroyed by an inflammatory process.

25 Mammography
Nodules with well-defined contours having the appearance of gross cysts.

26 Pneumocystography
This shows cystic cavities.

27 HES ×1
Mount section of FCD in which cysts are the dominant feature.

28 HES ×1
Mount section of a gross cyst opened at operation.

29 HES ×25
Gross cyst: fibrous wall without epithelial lining.

30 HES ×64
Ruptured cyst: the apocrine epithelium still visible on the edges is destroyed elsewhere and replaced by foamy histiocytes.

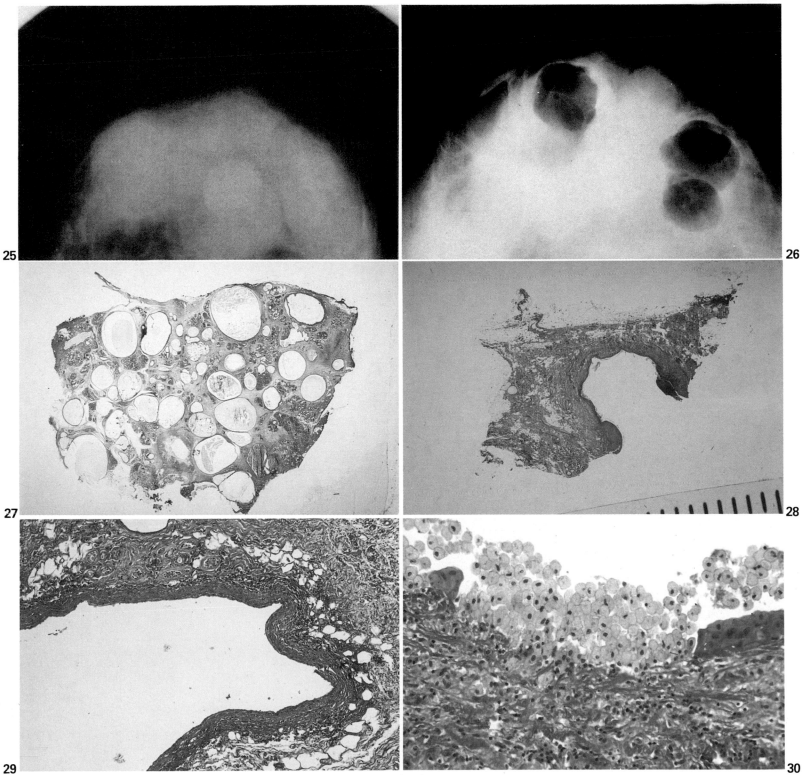

2.2 EPITHELIOSIS

Synonyms

Papillomatosis, ductal epithelial hyperplasia.

Definition

Abnormal multiplication of epithelial cells within pre-existing glandular structures, particularly extra and intralobular terminal ducts.

- Pathological criteria are valid only when taken together. Taken alone, none can confirm benignity.
- Differential diagnosis with ductal carcinoma in situ is sometimes difficult.
- Epitheliosis does not usually affect the subareolar major ducts. Such a diagnosis at this site is suspicious and corresponds more probably to a ductal carcinoma in situ.

---

31 HES ×25
Epitheliosis in an extralobular terminal duct.

32 HES ×10
Epitheliosis in ductules (or acini).

33 HES ×10
Epitheliosis in a major duct (rare feature).

34 HES ×25
Epitheliosis: *fenestrated* pattern with serpiginous splits.

35 HES ×64
Epitheliosis: *solid* pattern.

36 HES ×64
Epitheliosis: *'tufting'* pattern.

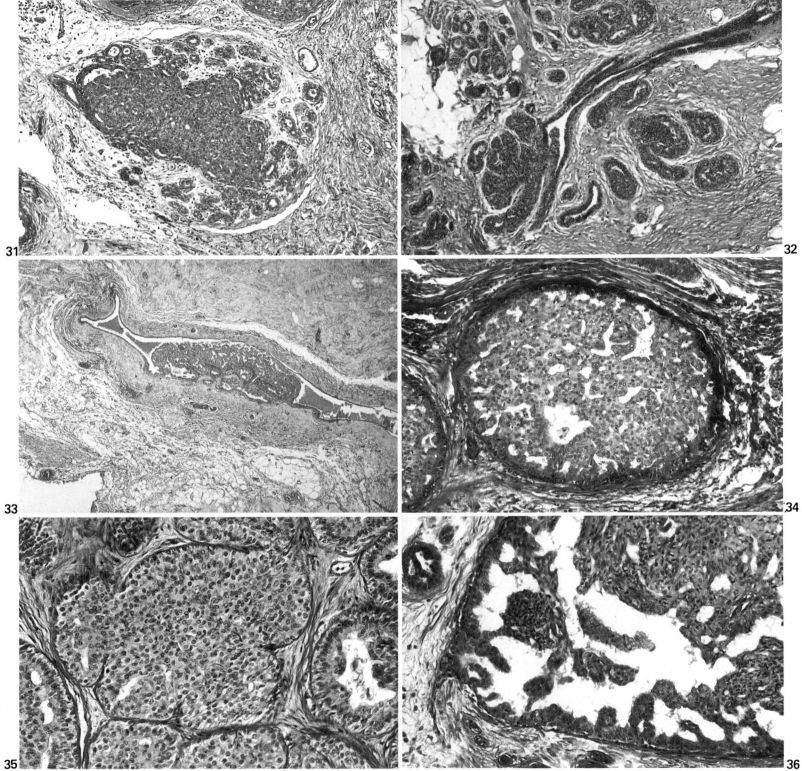

37 HES ×160
Epitheliosis: swirling of cells.

38 HES ×64
Epitheliosis: spindle cells arranged in fascicles or streaming pattern.

39 HES ×160
Epitheliosis: spindle-cell bridging with elongated cells arranged parallel to the long axis of the bridges.

40 HES ×64
Calcifications, rare feature in epitheliosis.

41 HES ×64
Epitheliosis: cells have ovoid nuclei without conspicuous nucleoli, indistinct cytoplasmic borders. In the centre, a cluster of foamy histiocytes.

42 HES ×160
Epitheliosis: frequency of pseudonucleoli.

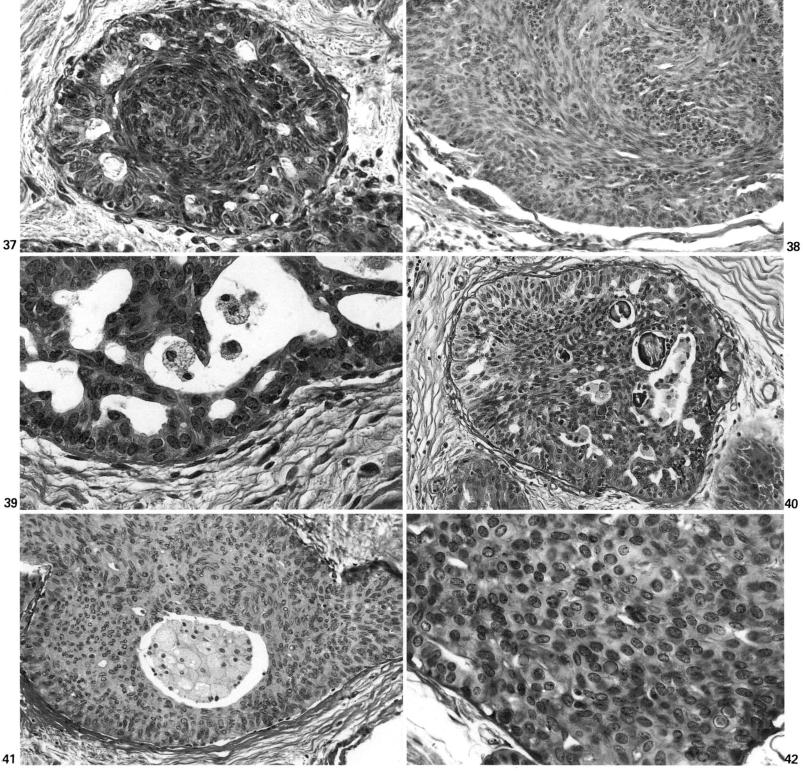

2.3 ADENOSIS

Synonym

Lobular epithelial hyperplasia.

Definition

Multiplication of the number of lobules with hyperplasia of all constituents (epithelial and myoepithelial cells, lobular stroma). This hyperplasia may be harmonious or one of the constituents may be predominant.

Variants

- simple
- sclerosing
- microglandular
- blunt duct adenosis

SIMPLE ADENOSIS

Lobules increase in size and multiply in number, but the lobular pattern is maintained. This may be real disease or simple accentuation of the normal structure under the influence of hormonal stimuli.

43 HES ×10
Simple adenosis.

44 HES ×10
Fibroadenomatous microfocus in diffuse lesion of adenosis: such areas without a real tumour are frequent in the fibrocystic disease of the breast. They develop in all or a part of the lobule.

SCLEROSING ADENOSIS

Synonyms

Nodular adenosis, tumour adenosis.

Definition

Lobular hyperplasia with distortion by stromal proliferation and fibrosis.

Pathology

- all degrees of distorted lobules are possible;
- *subgroups:* (i) sclerosing adenosis localized around extralobular terminal ducts
  (ii) involutive sclerosing adenosis of either myoid or fibrous type.

45 Mammography
Distortion of glandular trabeculae.

46 Surgical specimen
Small granular and whitish areas not typical of carcinoma.

47 HES ×1
A whole mount section shows a conglomeration of small nodules corresponding to lobules (responsible for the granular macroscopic aspect).

48 HES ×10
Lobules are quite disorganized but they are still surrounded by a collagen ring (persistence of lobular configuration). The architectural pattern here is very important.

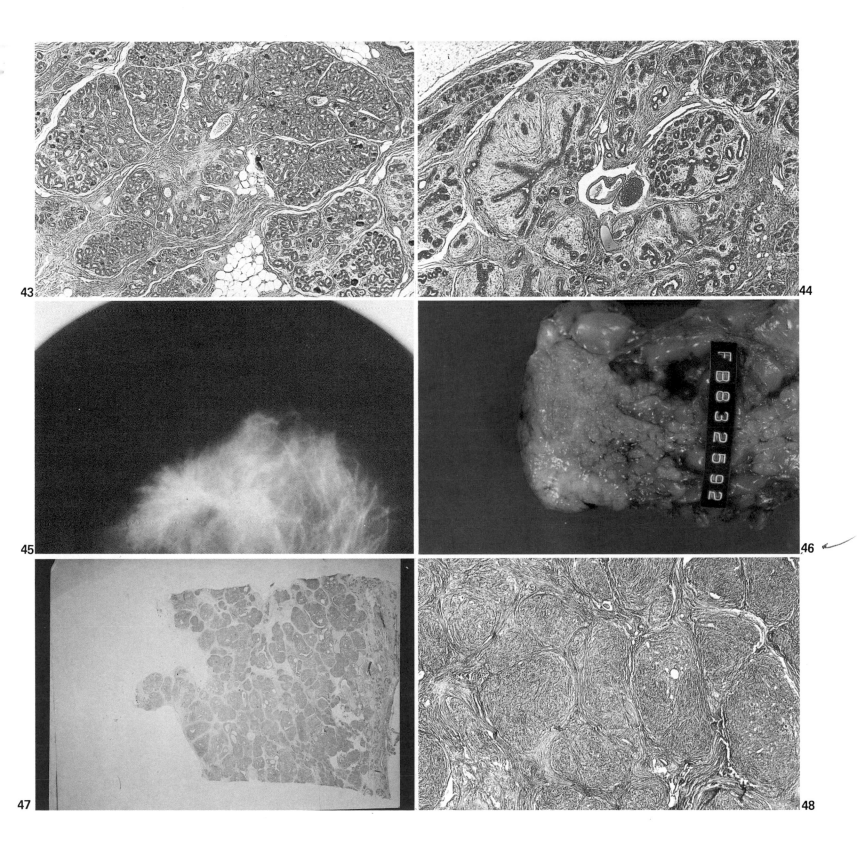

Danger of mistaking this lesion for carcinoma. The pathologist must not be influenced by suspect clinical and radiological features. Advice may be given to avoid errors:
- frozen sections: the size of the sample has to be sufficient. In case of doubtful diagnosis, wait for paraffin sections.
- paraffin sections: examination at low power magnification is essential because the criterion of benignity is sometimes only architectural (lobular pattern preserved).

All degrees of distortion within the lobule.

49 HES ×25
Interstitial fibrosis with persistent terminal ductules (acini).

50 HES ×25
Apocrine metaplasia.

51 HES ×25
Terminal ductules (acini) are compressed and distorted by fibrosis (not to be mistaken for IDC).

52 HES ×10
Terminal ductules (acini) persist as microtubules (not to be mistaken for a tubular carcinoma).

53 HES ×25
A lobule is disorganized but well circumscribed by sclerosis.

54 HES ×25
A disorganized lobule with sclerohyaline and elastosic areas.

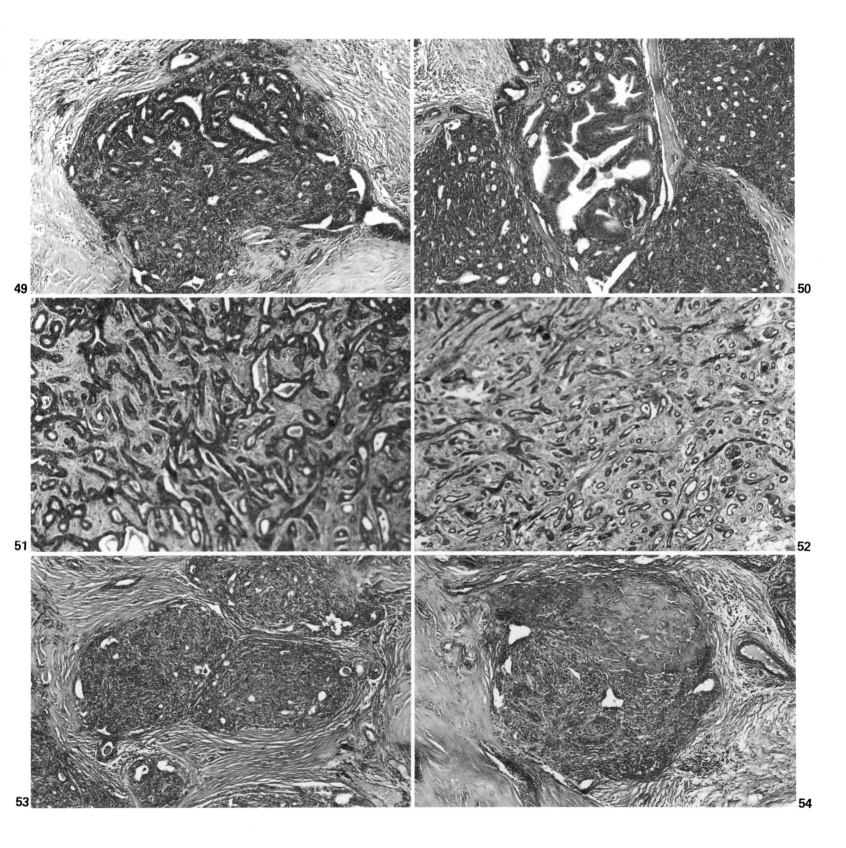

55 HES ×64

A few terminal ductules persist; the others have been destroyed and replaced by epithelial trabeculae separated by fibromyoid stroma.

56 S100 protein ×64

The stroma contains myoepithelial cells with myoid differentiation and is positive with S100 protein staining.

57 HES ×64
58 HES ×160
59 HES ×160
60 HES ×160

Rare terminal ductules persist with intraluminal calcifications. Large cells with round nuclei and abundant pale cytoplasm are scattered among other cells (not to be mistaken for a lobular carcinoma in situ or invasive).

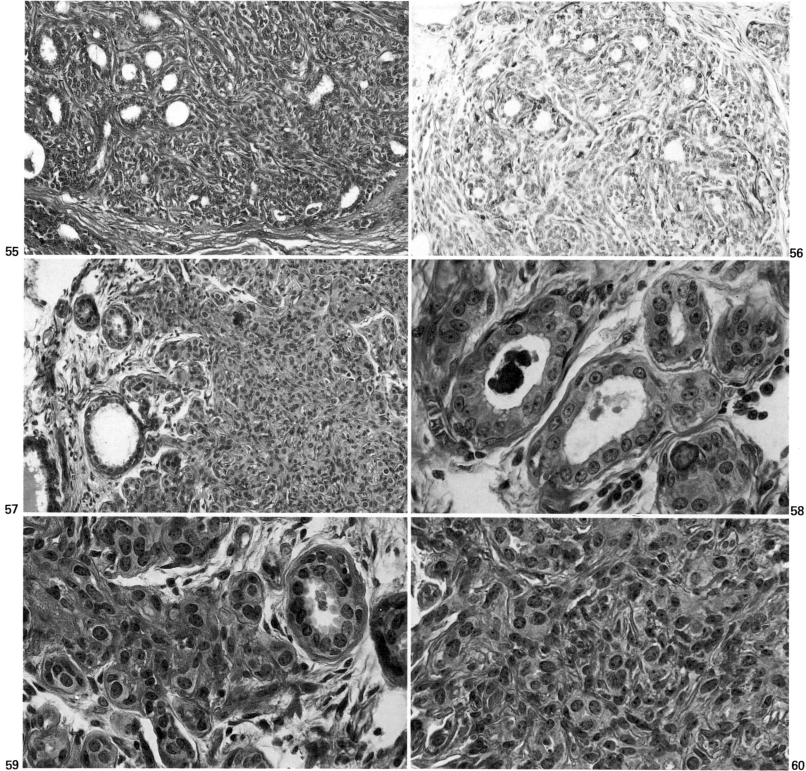

SCLEROSING ADENOSIS
Two subgroups

61 HES ×10
Pericanalicular sclerosing adenosis.
Particular site around extralobular terminal ducts (possibly of ductal rather than lobular origin).

62 HES ×64
Involutive sclerosing adenosis with myoid inflexion. Epithelial structures have almost totally disappeared. The myoepithelial component remains with a myoid differentiation.

63 HES ×25
64 HES ×64
Involutive sclerosing adenosis.
With sclerous inflexion: epithelial structures are disappearing. Sclerosis is predominant with a hyaline nodule punctuated by psammoma bodies.

MICROGLANDULAR ADENOSIS

Definition

Proliferation of small glands lying randomly in fibrous and adipose tissue without lobular arrangement (term proposed by McDivitt, Stewart and Berg in 1968).

> **Benign lesion with possible precancerous potential that can mimic a tubular carcinoma.**

65 HES ×25
66 HES ×64
Typical histological pattern of microtubules
- regular size and distribution without stroma reaction (as opposed to tubular carcinoma)
- opened lumina with a PAS-positive, diastase-resistant secretion
- a single cell layer (no myoepithelial cells)
- absence of apical snouts and trabecular bars bridging the lumina (as opposed to tubular carcinoma).

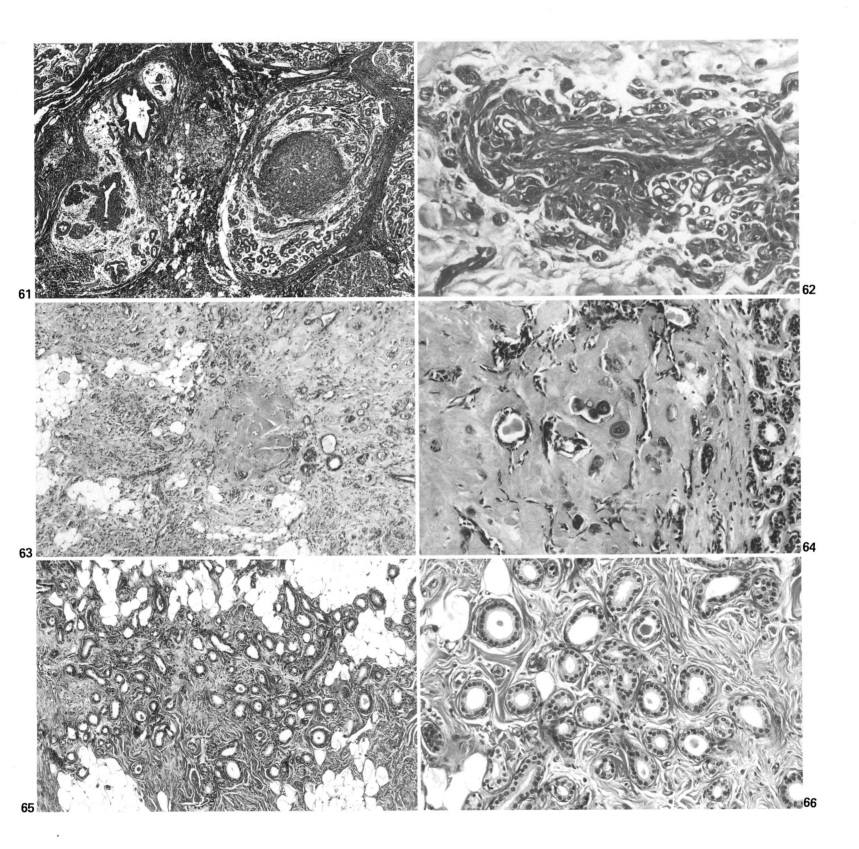

BLUNT DUCT ADENOSIS

Terminology

See Figure 84.

Definition

'Proliferation of small ducts which end abruptly and do not terminate in lobules. Blunted ducts usually originate at the distal extremities of the duct system' (term proposed by Foote and Stewart in 1945).

Pathology

The authors describe two progressive phases:
- an early phase characterized by ducts with a two-cell-layer epithelium and apical snouts (or cytoplasmic blebs).
- a late phase characterized by ducts with wide lumen and cuboidal flattened epithelium. The myoepithelial cell layer is scarcely visible or not visible at all. Lumen often contains a secretion product.
- an intermediate phase may be added, characterized by the presence of a double cell layer which is less hyperplastic and has no apical snouts.

Genesis

It is debated whether it develops either from extra-lobular terminal ducts or from pre-existing lobules.

- Lobular configuration of blind ducts, the stroma being of either intralobular type or common collagen;
- Frequent coexistence of early and late BDA in the same breast;
- Frequent coexistence with epitheliosis;
- Presence of calcifications within intraluminal pseudo-papillary vegetations;
- Possible role in genesis of cancer with continuum between blunt duct adenosis and ductal carcinoma in situ.

---

67 HES ×10
68 HES ×25
69 HES ×160
BDA early phase;
lobular configuration, hyperplasia of two cell layers, apical snouts.

70 HES ×64
BDA intermediary phase;
two cell layers, no apical snouts.

71 HES ×25
72 HES ×64
BDA late phase;
ducts with large lumen containing secretion and a single cell layer visible.

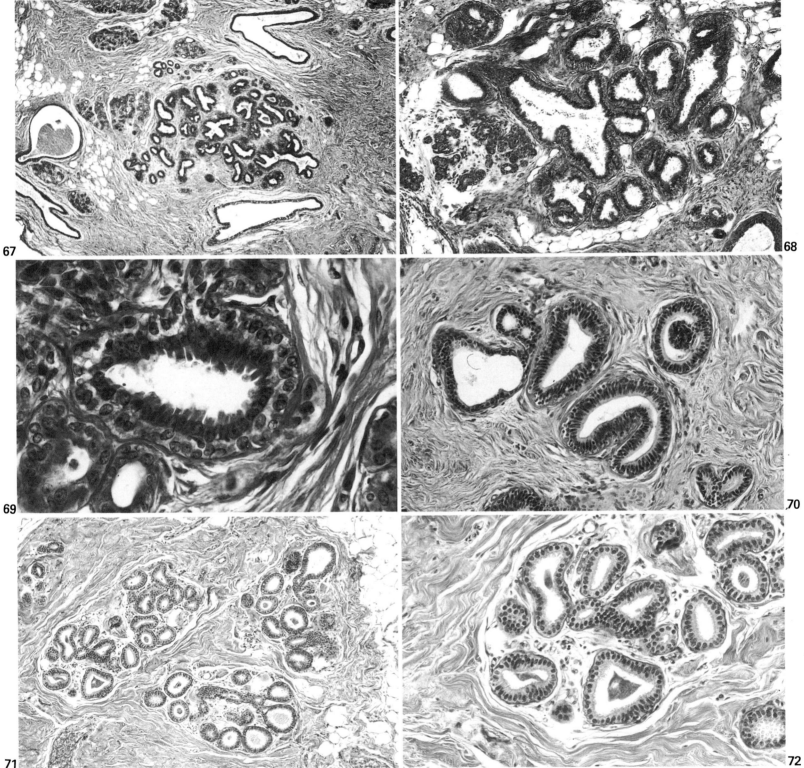

73 HES ×64
Calcification within an intraluminal pseudopapillary growth.

74 HES ×64
BDA within a nerve.

75 HES ×25
76 HES ×160
BDA with hyperplasia and myoid differentiation of myoepithelial cell layer.

77 HES ×25
78 HES ×64
Epitheliosis coexisting with BDA.

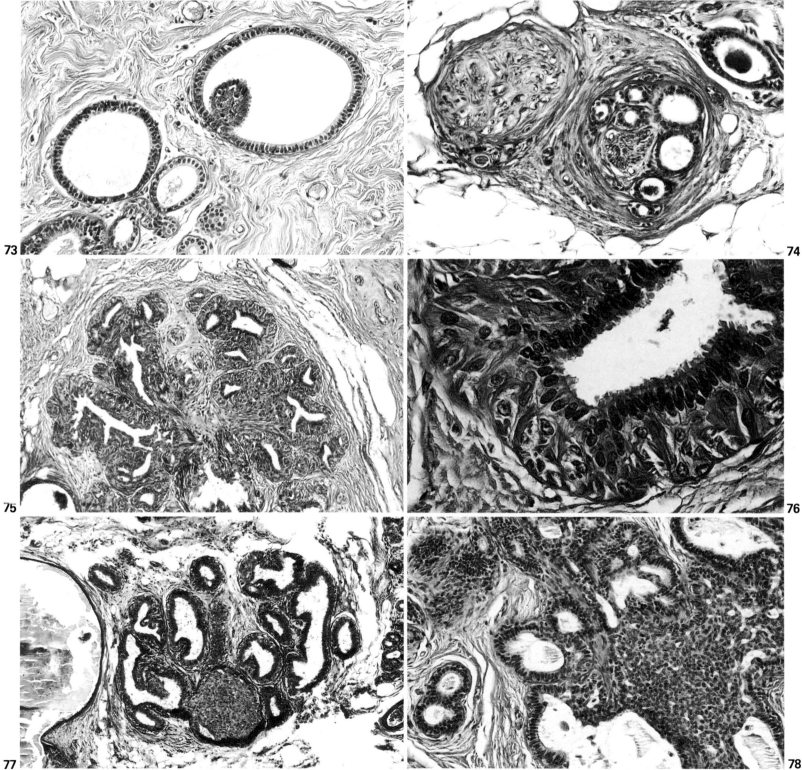

79 HES ×10
BDA, early phase.

80 Orcein ×10
Absence of elastic tissue around terminal ducts of BDA.

81 EMA ×10
Epithelial cell positivity in ducts and BDA, but weak or negative in acini.

82 Cytok ×10
Positivity of all epithelial cells (ducts, BDA, acini).

83 S100 Protein ×64
Positivity of myoepithelial cells in a duct of BDA.

84 Terminology of BDA.

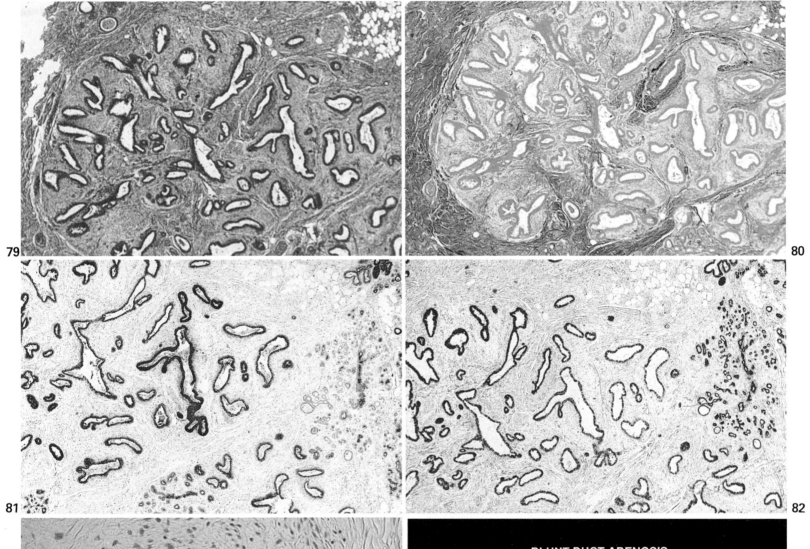

BONSER (1961)	FOOTE (1945) HAAGENSEN (1981)	WELLINGS (1975)	AZZOPARDI (1979)
Columnar	Blunt Duct Adenosis	Atypical lobule A	
metaplasia	early phase	grades I. II.II.	Blunt Duct Adenosis
	late phase	a few grades IV	
			Microcystic BDA
			Non-organoid BDA

BLUNT DUCT ADENOSIS

TERMINOLOGY

2.4 RADIAL SCAR

Synonyms

Sclerosing papillomatosis (Haagensen, 1968), infiltrating epitheliosis (Azzopardi, 1979), non-encapsulated sclerosing lesion (Fisher, 1979), indurative mastopathy (Rickert, 1981), Aschoff's proliferation centre (Contesso, 1985), sclerosing ductal proliferation (Tremblay, 1977).

The term 'radial scar' was adopted by Linell (1980).

Definition

Stellate formation with scleroelastosic centre towards which terminal ductal-lobular units radially converge.

Frequency

Depends on two factors:
1. higher if the number of examined blocks is greater.
2. histological context: radial scars are more often associated with malignant than with benign lesions (26% against, 14% respectively; Wellings, 1984).

Size

From 3 to 10mm, usually microscopic.
There are clinical and mammographic signs only for the largest ones.

85 Surgical specimen
Small stellate lesion (4mm) with a bluish cyst.

86 Diagram of elements implicated in the formation of the radial scar.

87 HES ×10 ⎫
88 Orcein ×10 ⎭
Radial scar, simple type.

89 HES ×5
Ductal obliterations at the edge of the radial scar.

90 HES ×25
Glands enclosed in the scleroelastosic centre are very elongated and distorted (to be distinguished from an invasive ductal carcinoma).

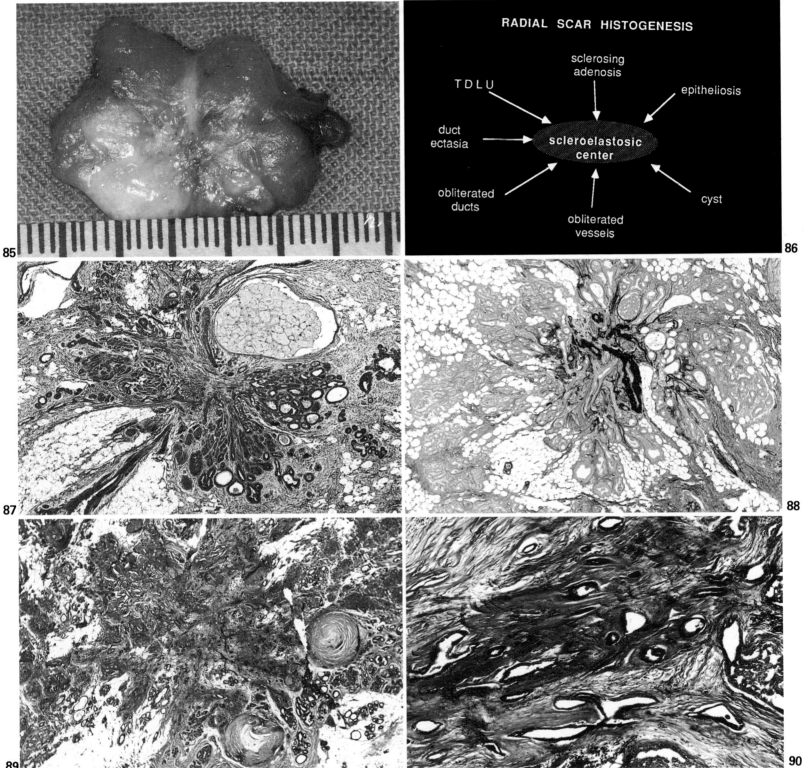

RADIAL SCAR HISTOGENESIS

TDLU

sclerosing
adenosis

epitheliosis

duct
ectasia

scleroelastosic
center

obliterated
ducts

obliterated
vessels

cyst

RADIAL SCAR AND EPITHELIOSIS

Histological types

- simple without any proliferative lesion, with some cysts,
- associated with proliferative lesions: epitheliosis, micropapillomas,
- associated with a cancer: lobular or ductal carcinoma in situ, tubular carcinoma.

For Linell, the first two types of carcinoma constitute an incidental finding since most of the carcinomas originate within the TDLU. Ductal carcinoma in situ and lobular carcinoma in situ may also be found outside the radial scar.

As for tubular carcinoma, Linell thinks it starts from the centre with centrifugal spreading. The scleroelastosic stroma should have a role as inductor of cancer, probably with other associated factors. However, not all authors agree with this view on the precancerous role of the radial scar.

Genesis

(See Figure 88) numerous factors (perhaps associative) are implicated.

- **Multicentric and bilateral lesion (multicentricity is correlated with the intensity of proliferative disease).**
- **Risk of error on frozen sections or conventional histological sections. In case of doubt, avoid the risk of excessive surgery on the patient.**
- **Frequent difficulty in diagnosing an early tubular carcinoma and in distinguishing epitheliosis from ductal carcinoma in situ.**

---

91 HES ×5
92 HES ×25
93 HES ×25
Radial scar with peripheral regular epitheliosis and micropapilloma.

94 HES ×25
Epitheliosis within the scleroelastosic centre.

95 HES ×25
96 HES ×64
Atypical epitheliosis. To be differentiated from a ductal carcinoma in situ.

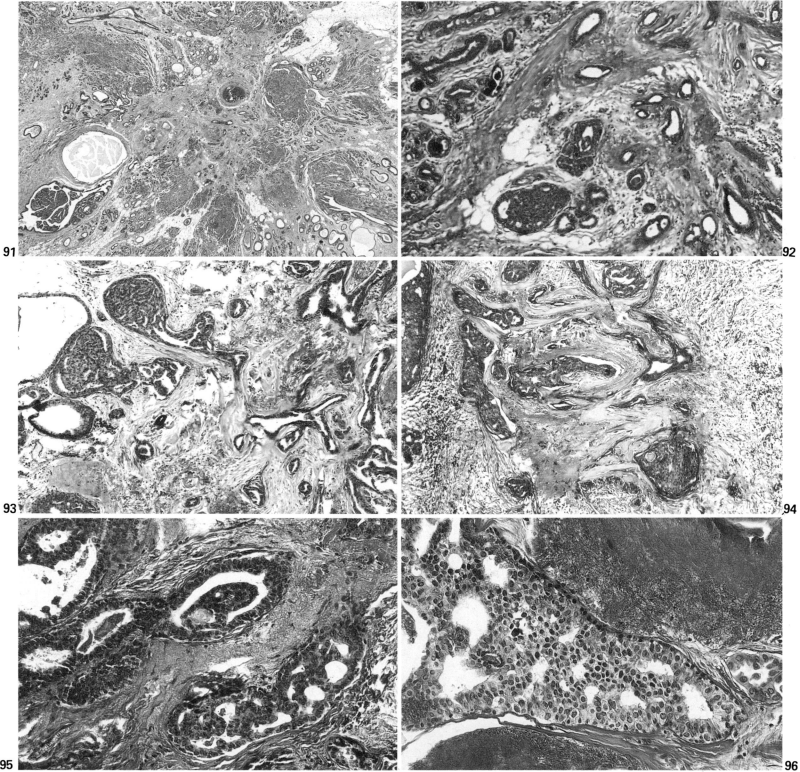

RADIAL SCAR AND CANCER

97 HES ×5 ⎫
98 HES ×64 ⎭
Radial scar with ductal carcinoma in situ (cribriform and bridging pattern) and epitheliosis.

99 HES ×5 ⎫
100 HES ×64 ⎭
Radial scar and early tubular carcinoma in the centre with typical angulated tubules.

101 HES ×10 ⎫
102 HES ×64 ⎭
Radial scar and lobular carcinoma in situ.

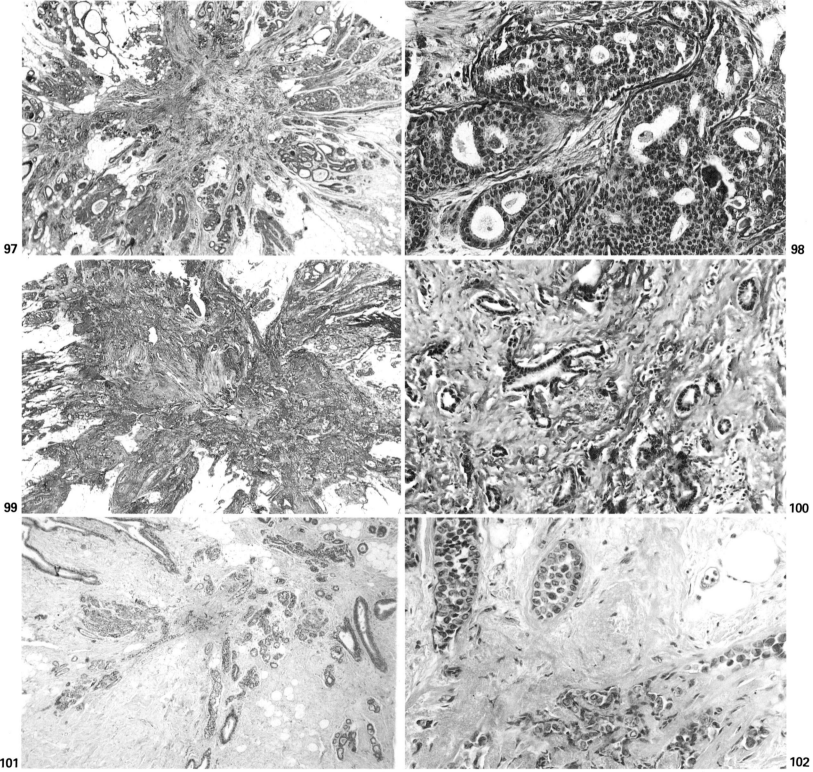

References
Chap. 2 – Fibrocystic Disease

Andersen, J.A. *et al.* (1984) Radial scar in the female breast. *Cancer*, **53**, 2557.

Azzopardi, J.G. (1983) Benign and malignant proliferative epithelial lesions of the breast; a review. *Eur. J. Cancer. Clin. Oncol.*, **19**, 1717.

Bonser, G.M. *et al.* (1961) Human and Experimental Breast Cancer, London: Pitman Medical.

Clement, P.B. *et al.* (1983) Microglandular adenosis of the breast, a lesion simulating tubular carcinoma. *Histopathology*, **7**, 169.

D'Amore, E. *et al.* (1985) Le centre prolifératif d'Aschoff. *Ann. Pathol.*, **5**, 173.

Dupont, W.D. *et al.* (1985) Risk factors for breast cancer in women with proliferative breast disease. *N. Engl. J. Med.*, **312**, 146.

Fisher, E.R. *et al.* (1983) Scar cancers: pathologic findings from the National Surgical Adjuvant Breast Project (Protocol N° 4)-IX-*Breast Cancer Res. Treat.*, **3**, 39.

Haagensen, D.E. *et al.* (1979) Breast gross cystic disease fluid analysis: isolated and radioimmunoassay for a major component protein. *J.N.C.I.*, **62**, 239.

Hutchinson, W.B. *et al.* (1980) Risk of breast cancer in women with benign breast disease. *J.N.C.I.*, **65**, 13.

Hutter, R.V.P. (1985) Goodbye to 'fibrocystic disease'. *N. Engl. J. Med.*, **312**, 179.

Love, S.M. *et al.* (1982) Fibrocystic 'disease' of the breast. A non disease? *N. Engl. J. Med.*, **307**, 1010.

Mascarel, I. *et al.* (1984) Analyse de 1225 exérèses mammaires partielles à visée diagnostique. Incidence de cancer et contexte histologique. *Bull. Cancer* (Paris), **71**, 425.

Mazoujian, G. *et al.* (1983) Immunohistochemistry of a gross cyst disease fluid protein (GCDFP-15) of the breast. *Am. J. Pathol.*, **110**, 105.

Page, D.L. (1986) Cancer risk assessment in benign breast biopsies. *Hum. Pathol.*, **17**, 875.

Rickert, R.R. *et al.* (1981) Indurative mastopathy. *Cancer*, **47**, 561.

Rosen, P.P. (1983) Microglandular adenosis. A benign lesion simulating invasive mammary carcinoma. *Am. J. Surg. Pathol.*, **7**, 137.

Tremblay, G. *et al.* (1977) Elastosis in benign sclerosing ductal proliferation of the female breast. *Ann. J. Surg. Pathol.*, **1**, 155.

Wellings, S.R. *et al.* (1984) Subgross pathologic features and incidence of radial scars in the breast. *Hum. Pathol.*, **15**, 475.

3
Papilloma

Papillomas are proliferative lesions of the ductal epithelium with a partial or total papillary pattern.

Papillae are defined by a fibrovascular core covered with an epithelial layer.

Several types of papillomas are distinguished:

- solitary intraductal papilloma
- multiple intraductal papilloma
- juvenile multiple intraductal papilloma
- microscopic papilloma
- papillary adenoma of the nipple

The division is a little artificial and these categories constitute only multiple facets of the proliferative breast disease, with their own respective characteristic features.

3.1 SOLITARY INTRADUCTAL PAPILLOMA

Synonyms

Papillary cystadenoma, central papilloma.

Definition

Arborescent lesion growing within one or several adjacent large ducts. This lesion can reach a size sufficient to fill up the duct, and thus become grossly visible, and sometimes give a palpable lump.

Clinical features

- All ages (mean age: 48 years).
- Serous or bloody nipple discharge (70%).
- Site: major collecting ducts in the subareolar area including milk sinuses.

Histological features

- Predominant papillary but also adenomatous or solid pattern.
- Changes: sclerosis, calcifications, apocrine metaplasia, infarction, hemorrhage.
- One duct or several contiguous ducts may be involved but usually not the TDLU.

No frozen sections of any papillary lesion (risk of erroneous diagnosis of carcinoma).

103 Galactography
Lacunar image in the duct.

104 Macroscopy
Small friable pedonculated tumour in the lumen of a duct.

105 HES ×5
A papilloma is free within the lumen of a dilated duct.

106 HES ×64
Papillary pattern: papillae have a fibrovascular core covered with an inner layer of myoepithelial cells and an outer layer of epithelial cells.

107 HES ×64 ⎫
108 HES ×64 ⎭
Adenomatous structure: the glandular structures are separated by a fibromyoid stroma, the lumina are full of foamy histiocytes.

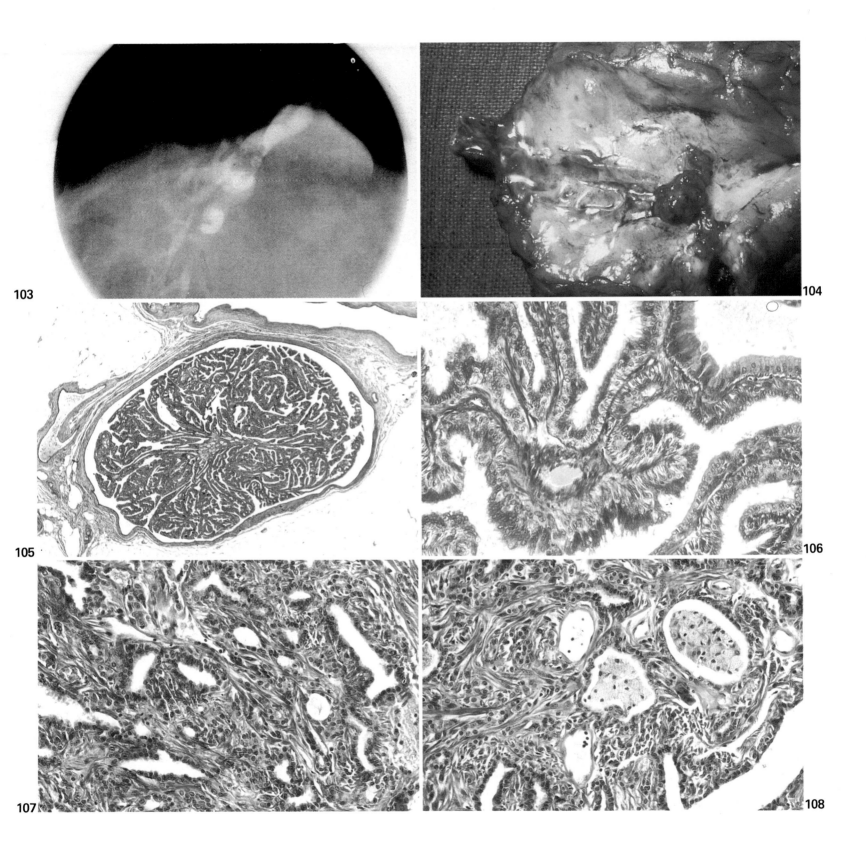

109 HES ×25
110 HES ×64
Solid epithelial hyperplasia of the epithelium of papillae.

111 HES ×25
Apocrine metaplasia.

112 HES ×25
The centres of the branches are modified by sclerosis, calcifications and foamy histiocytes.

113 HES ×25
Fibrous distortion at the site of implantation, that may have a pseudocarcinomatous aspect.

114 HES ×5
Massive infarction of a papilloma.

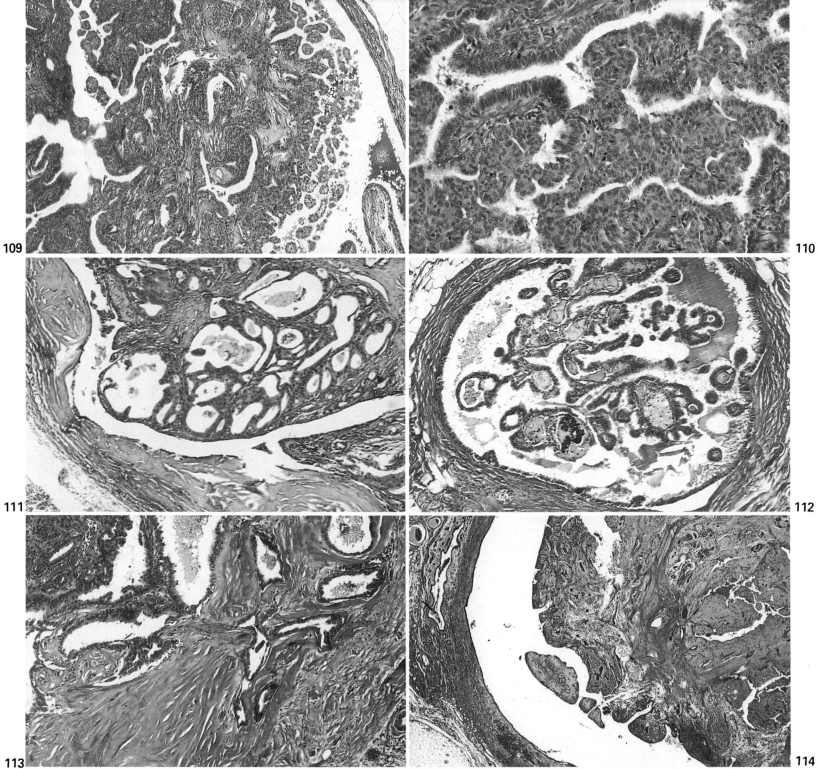

3.2 MULTIPLE INTRADUCTAL PAPILLOMA

Synonym

Peripheral papilloma.

Definition

Arborescent papillary and multifocal lesion, with a palpable tumour.

Clinical features

- Earlier age than for solitary papilloma (mean age: 40 years).
- Nipple discharge in 20% of cases.
- Often bilateral and recurring.
- Site: distal and multifocal.

Histological features

- mixed pattern with frequent solid areas,
- changes: sclerosis, squamous metaplasia,
- have always a root in the TDLU but can spread into the large ducts,
- possible association with a ductal carcinoma in situ. This association may be due to a malignant change of papilloma or only to coexistence at the same site (most of the carcinomas start in the TDLU).

115 Orcein ×10 ⎫
116 HES ×64 ⎭
Root of a multiple papilloma in the TDLU; the extra-lobular duct is surrounded by elastic tissue which disappears in the lobule.

117 HES ×10 ⎫
118 HES ×10 ⎭
Multiple papilloma with fibrous distortion and pseudocarcinomatous aspect.

119 HES ×25
Multiple papilloma: site in a small duct.

120 HES ×64
Squamous metaplasia in a papilloma.

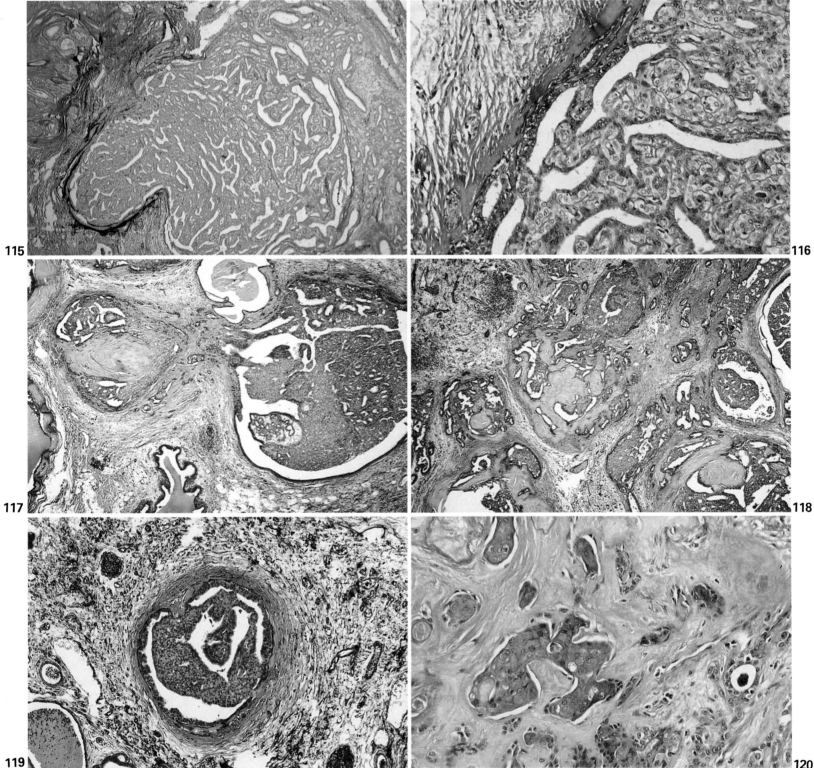

MALIGNANT CHANGE OF A MULTIPLE PAPILLOMA
IN DUCTAL CARCINOMA IN SITU

121 HES ×25 ⎫
122 HES ×64 ⎭
Benign papilloma with papillae covered with two cell layers.

123 HES ×64
Small area of DCIS in the papilloma.

124 HES ×25
A few adenomatous structures remain, gradually destroyed by the DCIS.

125 HES ×64
Typical cribriform pattern of DCIS.

126 HES ×64
Away from the papilloma, presence of 'lobular cancerization' with cribriform pattern in one acinus.

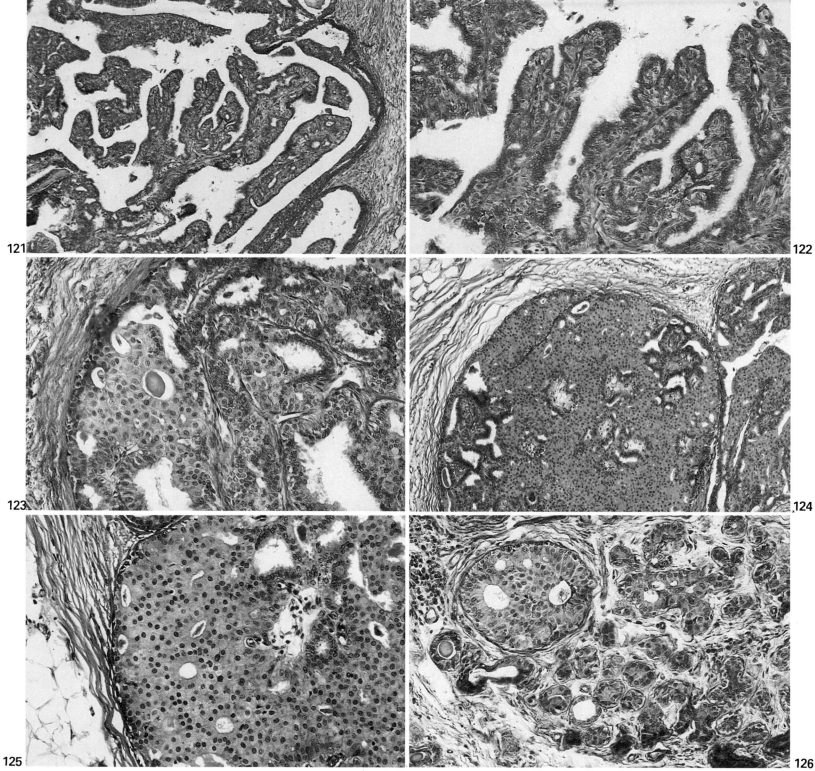

3.3 JUVENILE MULTIPLE INTRADUCTAL PAPILLOMA

Synonym

Juvenile papillomatosis.

Nosology

This lesion could be classified in fibrocystic disease. It tends to prove that papillary lesions are an integral part of proliferative disease of the breast.

Definition

This lesion is defined by the association of the following criteria (as opposed to classical FCD).

- The young age of the patients (20 years).
- Localized palpable tumour and unilateral character.
- Predominance of cysts and papillary apocrine metaplasia with areas of atypical epithelial hyperplasia and necrosis.

This lesion is considered benign but its precancerous potential is debated (Rosen, P.P.).

127 HES ×5
128 HES ×10

Histological appearances similar to those of the FCD: foci of epitheliosis and numerous cysts with papillary apocrine metaplasia.

3.4 MICROSCOPIC PAPILLOMA

This papilloma is not really an individualized entity. It is similar to a macroscopic papilloma and is distinguished from it only by its very small size. It can be found everywhere in the duct system but is more frequent at a distal level in the TDLU where it often coexists with epitheliosis. Apocrine or not, it only represents, like epitheliosis, one element of proliferative disease of the breast. Some authors think there is a continuum between epitheliosis and micropapillomas, and that the epithelial hyperplasia could turn from the solid structure of epitheliosis into a papillary structure when it develops in larger ducts. Epitheliosis would be thus a prepapillomatous stage.

129 HES ×10
130 HES ×25

Intrication at a distal level of solid epithelial hyperplasia (epitheliosis) and papillary hyperplasia (micropapilloma).

131 HES ×10
132 HES ×25

Intrication of adenosis and microscopic papilloma.

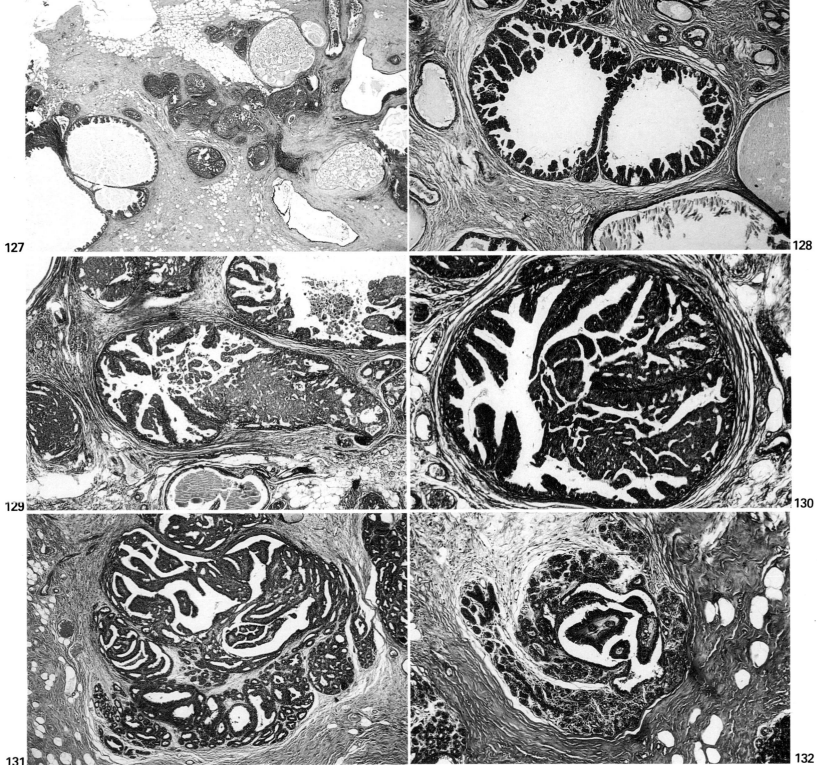

3.5 PAPILLARY ADENOMA OF THE NIPPLE

Synonyms

Florid papillomatosis of the nipple ducts, subareolar duct papillomatosis.

Definition

Benign proliferative lesion originating within a milk sinus and infiltrating diffusely through the nipple.

Clinical features

- all ages,
- it may mimic Paget's disease clinically,
- two evolutive stages:
  (i) pre-erosive stage with tumourous thickening and reddening of the nipple,
  (ii) erosive stage with a granuloma-like lesion on the nipple surface.

Histological features

A lesion which is both adenoid and papillary, not confined within the limits of a duct but diffusely infiltrating the substance of the nipple.

> - **Benign lesion without precancerous significance: malignant change is quite rare.**
> - **Erroneous diagnosis of carcinoma occurs frequently.**
> - **It is necessary to remove the entire tumour for diagnosis and not only a small superficial biopsy.**

Variant of nipple adenoma: syringomatous adenoma of the nipple
Its genesis is debated: tumour of skin adnexal origin or fibrosed form of papillary adenoma of the nipple.

133 Clinical appearance
Nipple adenoma forming a bulge on the surface.

134 HES ×10
Infiltration of the nipple stroma.

135 HES ×64
Papillary formations with double cell layers.

136 HES ×64
Fenestrated epithelial hyperplasia with sclerosis.

137 HES ×64 ⎫
138 HES ×160 ⎭
Syringomatous adenoma with small double cell layer tubules infiltrating the nipple stroma.

References
Chap. 3 – Papilloma

Bazzochi, F. *et al.* (1986) Juvenile papillomatosis (epitheliosis) of the breast. *Am. J. Clin. Pathol.*, **86**, 745.

Flint, A. *et al.* (1984) Infarction and squamous metaplasia of intraductal papilloma. *Hum. Pathol.*, **15**, 764.

Ohuchi, N. *et al.* (1984) Origin and extension of intraductal papillomas of the breast. A 3-D reconstruction study. *Breast Cancer Res. Treat.*, **4**, 117.

Ohuchi, N. *et al.* (1984) Possible cancerous change of intraductal papillomas of the breast. A 3-D reconstruction study of 25 cases. *Cancer*, **54**, 605.

Ohuchi, N. *et al.* (1985) Three-dimensional atypical structure in intraductal carcinoma differentiating from papilloma and papillomatosis of the breast. *Breast Cancer Res. Treat.*, **5**, 57.

Papotti, M. *et al.* (1983) Immunohistochemical analysis of benign and malignant papillary lesions of the breast. *Am. J. Surg. Pathol.*, **7**, 451.

Perzin, K.H. *et al.* (1972): Papillary adenoma of the nipple. *Cancer*, **29**, 996.

Rosen, P.P. (1983) Syringomatous adenoma of the nipple. *Am. J. Surg. Pathol.*, **7**, 739.

Rosen, P.P. (1985) Papillary duct hyperplasia of the breast in children and young adults. *Cancer*, **56**, 1611.

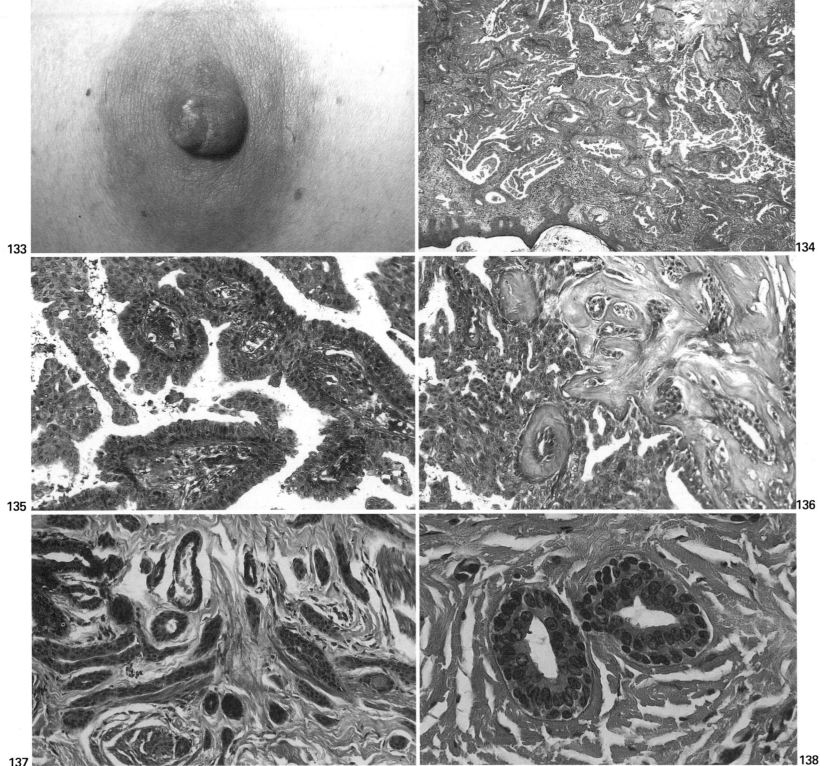

4

Duct ectasia

Synonyms

Varicocele tumour, periductal mastitis, plasma cell mastitis, comedomastitis, mastitis obliterans.

Definition

Inflammatory lesion characterized by the dilatation of the ducts, fibrosis and inflammation around them. It mainly concerns large ducts beneath the nipple and areola, and can be segmental or spread towards medium or small ducts.

There are several progressive stages each one having its own particular pathological, clinical and radiological features (Figure 139). Furthermore, there may be an infraclinical stage corresponding to a moderate ductal dilatation.

Etiology
- essential (often detected at operation for another lesion, fibrocystic disease or cancer). For Haagensen (1951), duct ectasia is 'a lesion of the inactive and ageing breast'.
- secondary to a papilloma or a DCIS.

Pathogenesis

It is debated whether primary dilatation of the ducts with stasis is responsible for inflammation and fibrosis, or primary inflammatory disease of the ducts produces lymphatic obstruction and dilatation of ducts.

Clinical and radiological features
- Can give pseudocarcinomatous aspects, clinically and radiologically.
- Nipple discharge (20%).
- Nipple inversion (30%).
- Very characteristic calcifications: tubular, annular and linear.

Histological features: Figure 139

Differential diagnosis

Is difficult with cysts and other inflammatory disorders.

4.1 DUCT ECTASIA: EARLY PHASE

This stage is characterized by dilated ducts, surrounded by a discrete or moderate inflammatory infiltrate.

139 Diagram of evolutive stages of duct ectasia correlations with clinical and radiological features.

140 Mammography
Spontaneously visible dilated ducts.

141 Mammography
Visibility of retroareolar ducts and nipple inversion.

142 Mount section
Simple duct ectasia in an old woman's atrophic breast.

143 HES ×5
Dilated duct with periductal lymphocytic infiltrate and eosinophilic amorphous debris.

144 HES ×25
Duct ectasia of an extralobular terminal duct.

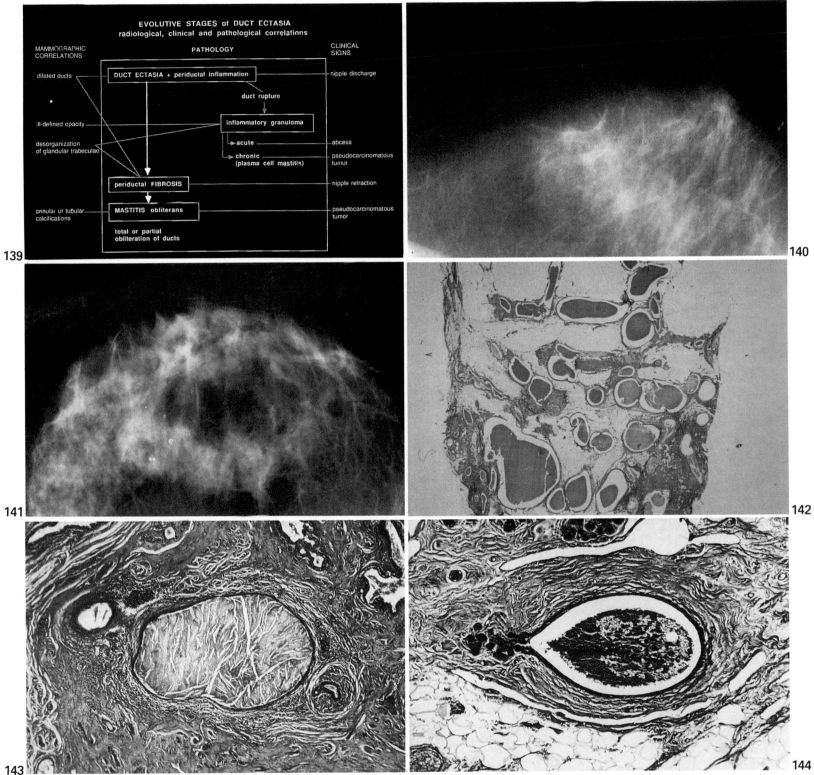

EVOLUTIVE STAGES of DUCT ECTASIA
radiological, clinical and pathological correlations

MAMMOGRAPHIC CORRELATIONS

PATHOLOGY

CLINICAL SIGNS

dilated ducts — DUCT ECTASIA + periductal inflammation — nipple discharge

duct rupture

ill-defined opacity — inflammatory granuloma

desorganization of glandular trabeculae

→ acute — abcess

→ chronic (plasma cell mastitis) — pseudocarcinomatous tumor

periductal FIBROSIS — nipple retraction

annular or tubular calcifications — MASTITIS obliterans — pseudocarcinomatous tumor

total or partial obliteration of ducts

139

140

141

142

143

144

4.2 DUCT ECTASIA: EVOLUTION TO FIBROSIS

The lesion can develop slowly into fibrosis until the late stage of complete ductal obliteration.

145 Mammography (fibrous stage)
Pseudocarcinomatous appearance with nipple inversion, skin thickening, retro-areolar dense image with short spicules extending in depth.

146 Surgical specimen (in Bouin's fixative liquid)
Ducts with dilated lumen surrounded by a dense opaque collar.

147 HES ×25
Large and regularly thick fibrous corona; lumen containing fatty debris.

148 HES ×25
Irregularly thick fibrous corona.

149 HES ×64
Radial structure of a crystalline body within intraductal material.

150 HES ×10
Duct with sinuous contours and shrinking of lumen due to a segmental fibrosis. Note the thick collar of elastic tissue at the edge of the fibrosis.

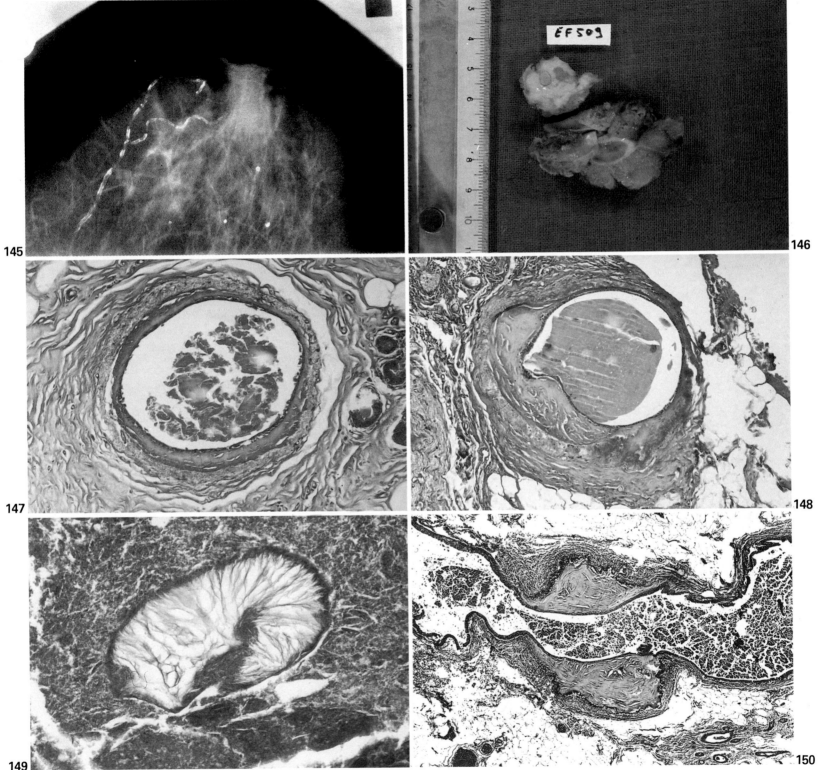

145

146

147

148

149

150

151 HES ×25
152 Orcein ×25

'Garland' pattern: the lumen of the duct is obliterated by a fibrous nodule. The 'garland' pattern is due to production of epithelium at the periphery of this nodule, in areas where it is not adherent to the duct wall. Note the periductal elastic tissue well visible by usual and specific stains.

153 HES ×25
154 Orcein ×25

'Garland' pattern associated with an inflammatory process. Foamy histiocytes fill the lumen of the transformed duct and lie outside the wall. The elastic coat is thinner and pushed back by the inflammatory infiltrate.

4.3 DUCT ECTASIA: END STAGE OF FIBROSIS: TOTAL OBLITERATION OF DUCTS

155 HES ×25

Contours of an obliterated duct with hyperelastosis. The centre is occupied by an oedematous fibrosis with two small glandular structures. Perhaps, they might represent a 'recanalization' similar to that of a thrombus.

156 HES ×25

Fibrous tissue totally obliterates the duct with disappearance of the epithelial lining. Elastic tissue outlines the original ductal contours.

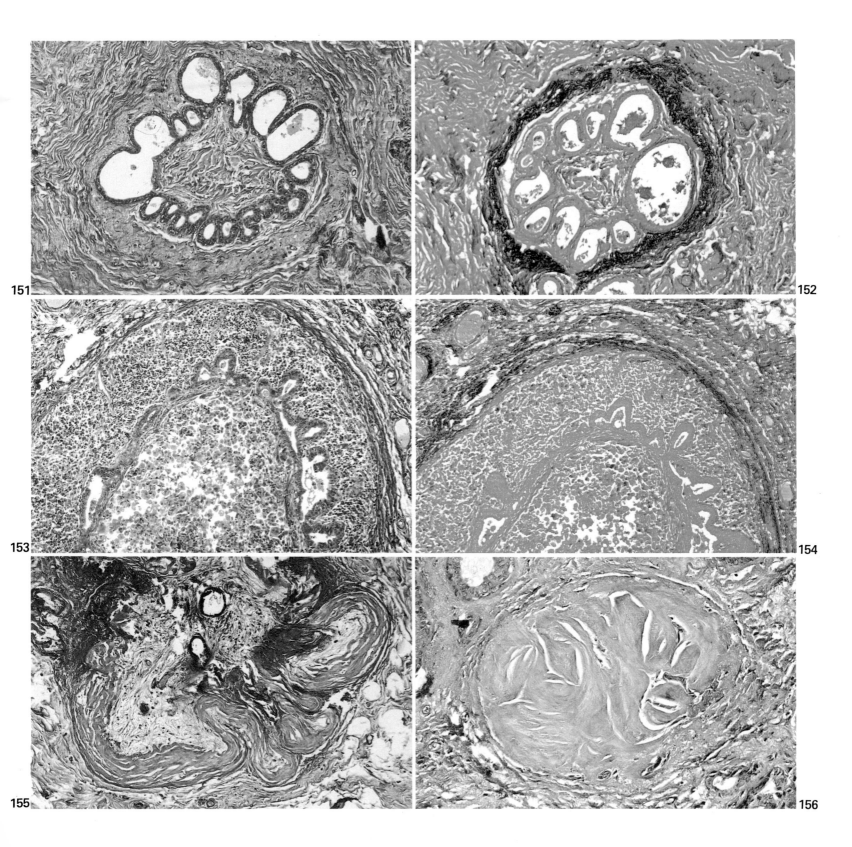

151

152

153

154

155

156

4.4 DUCT ECTASIA: EVOLUTION TO INFLAMMATION:
PLASMA CELL MASTITIS

The lesion can develop into a major inflammation with rupture of the duct wall. The lipid material gets into the periductal tissue. The inflammatory reaction shows sometimes a predominance of plasma cells (so-called plasma cell mastitis).

157 Mammography
Nodular opacity with ill-defined contours.

158 HES ×25
A duct being destroyed; lumen is still visible with a small area of vestigial epithelium.

159 Orcein ×25
Periductal elastic tissue is being destroyed.

160 HES ×64
Pleomorphic granuloma with phagocytic giant cells and a histiocytic lining around the lumen of the destroyed duct.

4.5 DUCT ECTASIA AND CANCER

Duct ectasia is often associated with cancer, but it is an incidental finding correlated with the high frequency of both lesions in the same age group.

161 HES ×25
Total obliteration of ducts, within an IDC.

162 HES ×10
Total obliteration of a duct; carcinomatous structures infiltrate the obliterated duct.

References
Chap. 4 – Duct Ectasia

Gershon-Cohen, J. *et al.* (1952) Secretory disease and plasma cell mastitis in the female breast. *Surg. Gynecol. Obstet.*, **95**, 497.

Haagensen, C.D. (1951) Mammary duct ectasia. *Cancer*, **4**, 749.

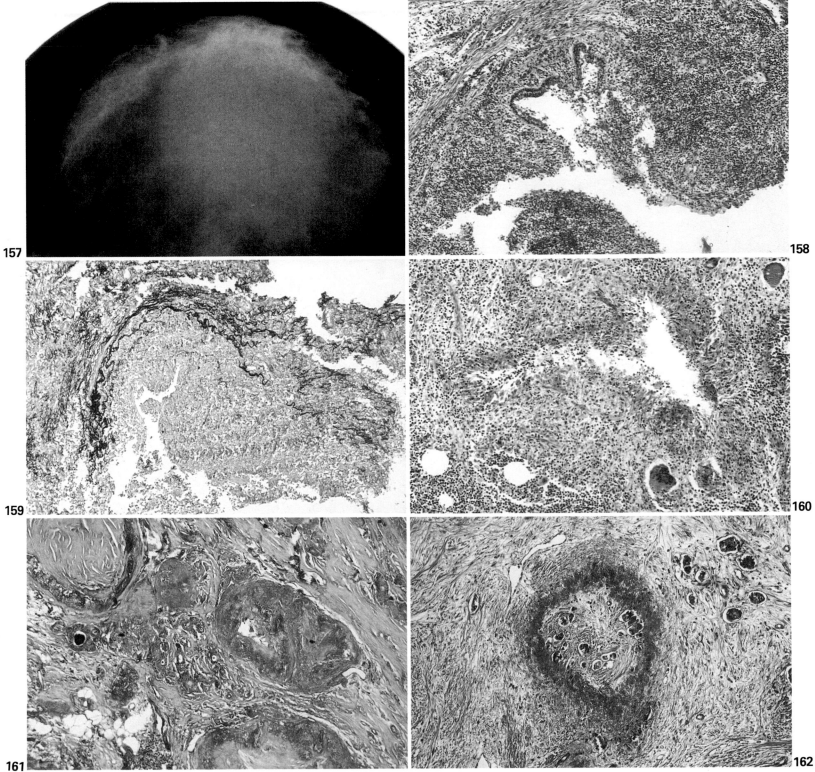

5
Fibroepithelial tumours

Tumours characterized by a proliferation of both epithelial and stromal component. They originate from the lobule and mainly include:

5.1 Fibroadenoma

5.2 Phyllodes tumour (cystosarcoma phyllodes)

5.3 Carcinosarcoma

5.1 FIBROADENOMA

Definition

Benign fibroepithelial proliferation usually forming a palpable nodular tumour. However, fibroadenomatous microfoci may be multiple and located sometimes only in a part of the lobule.

Clinical features

- all ages, all sizes, uni- or bilateral, solitary or multiple.
- may:
  - (i) recur
  - (ii) change to phyllodes tumour (whose progressive potential is uncertain)
  - (iii) contain a carcinoma (most often lobular in situ).

Therefore, excision appears to be justified.

Radiological features: Figures 163–164.

Macroscopic features: Figures 165–166.

Histological features

163 Nodular opacity with a sharp outline, surrounded by a translucent zone.

164 Multiple nodules with sharp outline, some of them are punctuated with large irregular calcifications.

165 Well-circumscribed nodule, soft and translucent.

166 Well-circumscribed nodule, firm and multilobulated.

TYPICAL FINDINGS

167 HES ×10
Pericanalicular type constituted of regular ducts.

168 HES ×10
Intracanalicular type: ducts are elongated, tortuous, distorted, presenting long clefts with a virtual lumen.

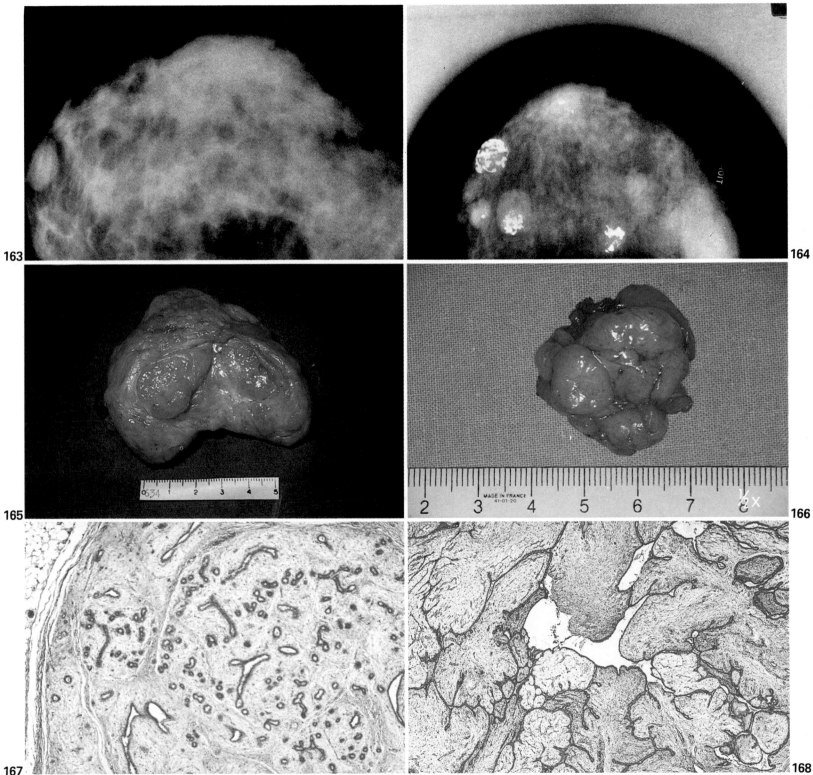

163
164
165
166
167
168

169 HES ×25
Appearance of a 'bouquet'. The stroma consists of fibroblasts within a loose stroma.

170 HES ×25
Mixed intra and pericanalicular type; a long cleft with a virtual lumen.

COMMON ASPECTS WITH THE PHYLLODES TUMOUR

171 HES ×10
Glandular lumen distorted but dilated with some polypoid projections (more frequent in phyllodes tumour).

172 HES ×25
Leaf-like appearance: fibroblasts and collagen have an arrangement like the veins of a leaf (also found in phyllodes tumours).

CHANGES

Concerning

- epithelial structures (frequent apocrine metaplasia, rare squamous metaplasia, secretory lobules, epithelial hyperplasia),
- the stroma (sclerosis, hyalinization, calcifications, myxoid change, rarely osteoid, chondroid or smooth muscle metaplasia), or
- both epithelium and stroma (sclerosing or microglandular adenosis, infarction).

173 HES ×10
Stromal sclerosis.

174 HES ×10
Myxoid stroma.

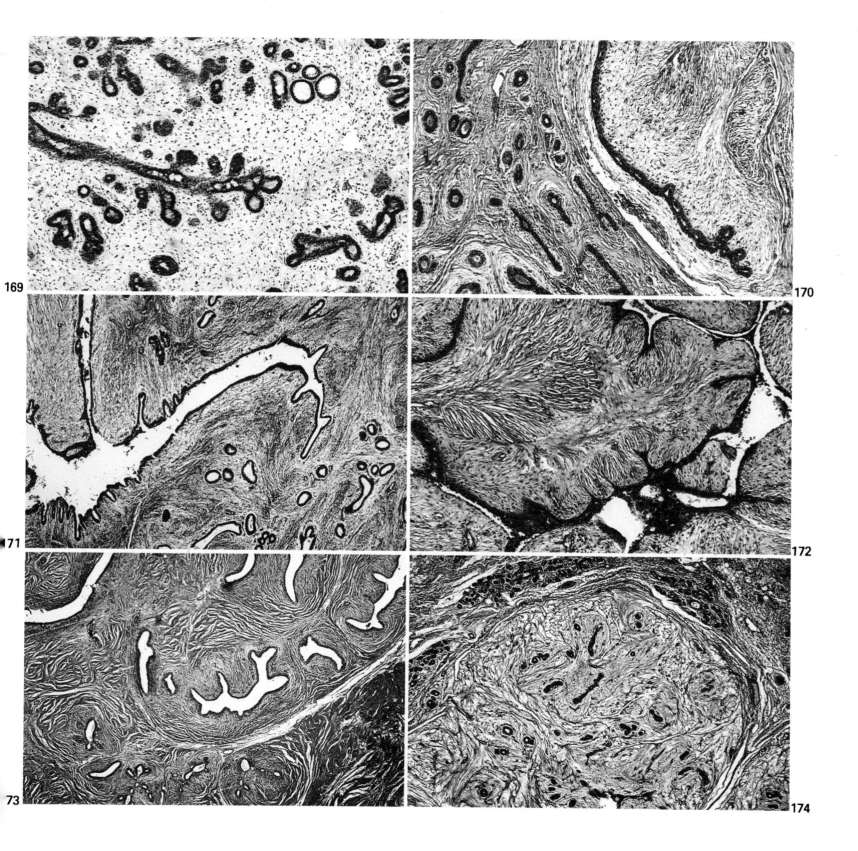

175 HES ×25
Area of sclerosing adenosis.

176 HES ×10
Secretory change in a fibroadenoma.

VARIANTS

Tubular adenoma and lactating adenoma

Nosology is questionable: Are tubular adenoma and lactating adenoma the same tumour? In this case, are they a variant of fibroadenoma affected by changes during pregnancy ('lactating'), or a separate entity with pure epithelial proliferation?

Here is an example of a giant fibroadenoma (12cm) of tubular type with secretory changes, revealed and operated on during pregnancy (4½ months).

177 Mammography
Dense opacity with sharp outline.

178 Gross pathology
Firm, multilobulated tumour.

179 HES ×5
Small tubular structures clustered in pseudolobules and separated by a scanty stroma.

180 HES ×160
Small tubules are lined by a prominent epithelial layer with cytoplasmic vacuolization. Nuclei have conspicuous nucleoli and myoepithelial cells are not visible.

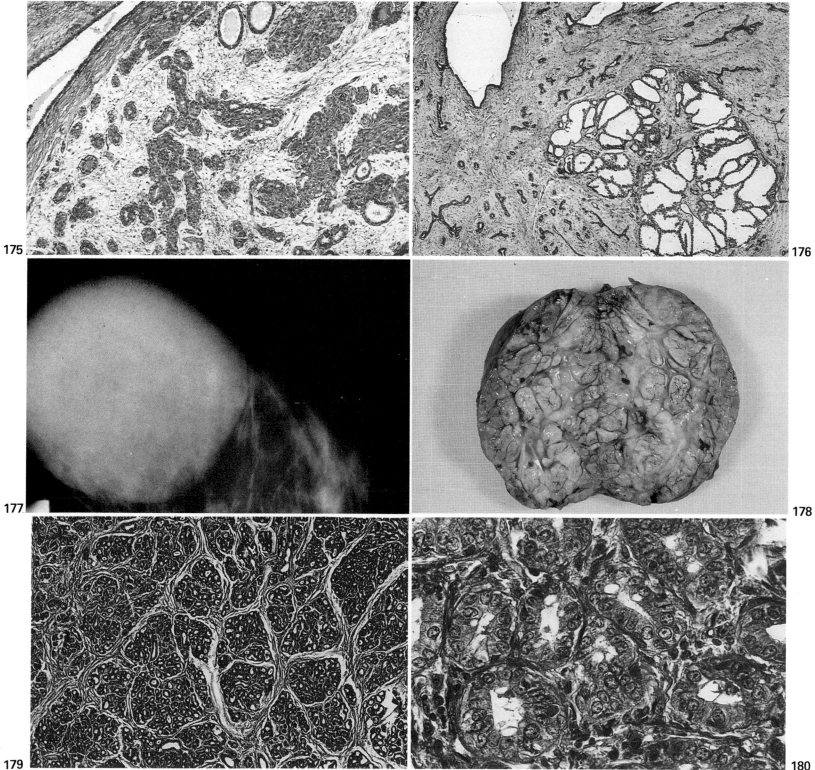

'Juvenile type' of fibroadenoma

The individualization of this variety (Ashikari, 1971) was based on the following criteria: 'benign fibroadenoma with cellular stroma and rapid growth in adolescent females'. It is actually the definition of the phyllodes tumour, which explains the variety of terms used (giant fibroadenoma, benign cystosarcoma phyllodes, cellular fibroadenoma). The criteria proposed to distinguish this tumour from a phyllodes tumour are (1) less stromal cellularity; (2) a predominant pericanalicular pattern.

This type of tumour has also been described, albeit uncommonly, in adults. In this case, the limits with a phyllodes tumour seem difficult to delineate.

Some fibroadenomas are also referred to as 'juvenile fibroadenomas' when the main feature is not an increased stromal cellularity but a severe atypical epithelial hyperplasia bordering on carcinoma in situ.

Fibroadenoma with pagetoid epithelial hyperplasia

The ductal epithelium is underlined by a hyperplastic layer of large cells with regular nuclei and clear cytoplasm. This hyperplasia looks like LCIS but without typical cytological characteristics. A similar lesion was termed by Azzopardi (1979) 'lobular endocrine neoplasia' in which the proliferative cells were of endocrine type.

181 HES ×10
182 HES ×64
Cellular stroma is constituted by regular fibroblasts with rare mitoses.

183 HES ×25
184 HES ×160
Pagetoid aspect: large clear cells underline the ductal epithelium (Grimelius negative).

FIBROADENOMA AND CANCER

Carcinoma arising in a fibroadenoma is very rare (about 1/1000). It may be restricted entirely to the fibroadenoma (originating in it), or also present in the adjacent tissues (secondary spread is then possible). It is most often a lobular carcinoma in situ.

185 HES ×10
186 HES ×25
The LCIS cells fill some of the epithelial crevices of fibroadenoma.

> Do not mistake a florid and exuberant but benign epithelial hyperplasia of some fibroadenomas for a ductal carcinoma in situ.

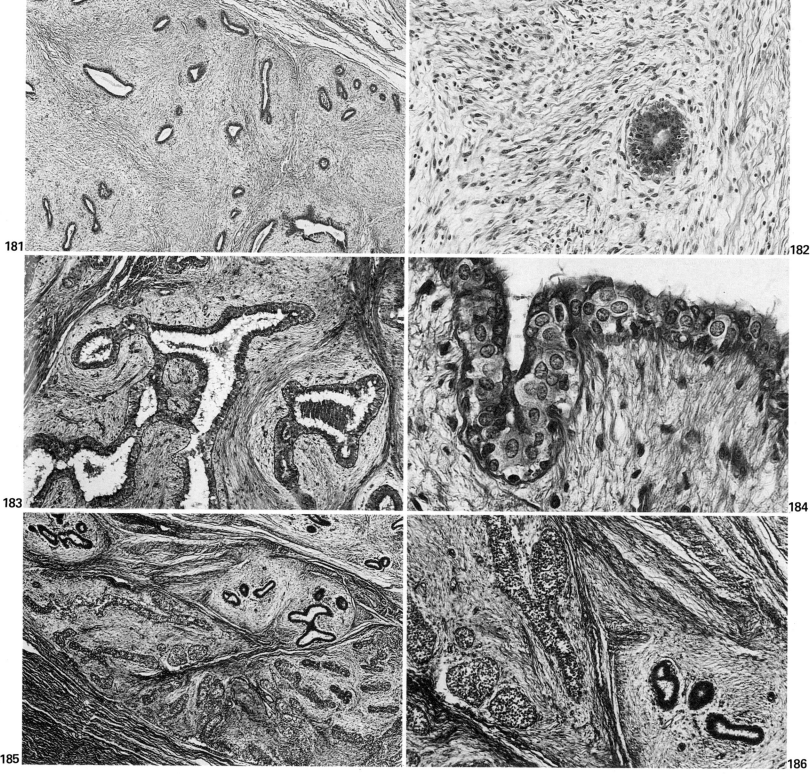

5.2 CYSTOSARCOMA PHYLLODES

Synonyms

Cellular intracanalicular fibroadenoma, fibroadenoma phyllodes, phyllodes tumour. 'Cystosarcoma phyllodes' is the name most frequently used but it is not satisfactory. Indeed, the word 'sarcoma' implies a malignant potential when most of these tumours are benign. A best designation would be 'phyllodes tumour'.

Definition

Fibroepithelial proliferation analogous to that of fibroadenoma but distinguished from it by stromal hypercellularity.

Clinical features

- mean age 45 years, exceptional at a young age,
- all sizes but most often large size, usually solitary and unilateral,
- rapid growth; skin ulceration is possible but does not indicate malignancy,
- *recurrence:* 20 to 30% of cases with the same pathological appearance (rarely increased malignancy),
- *metastases:* 3 to 12% of cases
  (i) anywhere
  (ii) always devoid of malignant epithelial component
  (iii) exceptional axillary node metastases.

Differential diagnosis between phyllodes tumour and fibroadenoma

- Heterogeneity (fibroadenoma is more homogeneous).
- Leaf-like pattern: not specific, also present in the intracanalicular type of fibroadenoma but with more narrow clefts and rare cystic formations (see Figures 171–172).
- Hypercellular and pleomorphic stroma: necrosis, sclerosis, various types of metaplasia (osseous, cartilaginous, adipous, smooth muscular).
- Epithelium, more often hyperplastic in phyllodes tumour than in fibroadenoma; squamous metaplasia frequent, apocrine metaplasia rare (as opposed to fibroadenoma).

Do not mistake epithelial hyperplasia for a ductal carcinoma in situ.

Genesis

From pre-existing fibroadenoma or de novo. Phyllodes tumours give rise to two pathological problems:
1. the differential diagnosis with fibroadenoma,
2. histoprognosis.

Gross pathology

Solid or most often partially cystic with intracystic vegetations.

187 Surgical specimen
The superior pole of the tumour consists of a solid area (histologically fibroadenoma) and the inferior pole consists of a cystic area containing a lobulated, gelatinous and translucent mass (histologically phyllodes tumour). This example supports the origin of phyllodes tumour from pre-existing fibroadenoma.

188 Surgical specimen
Vegetations resembling grape clusters protrude in a cystic cavity.

189 HES ×25
Ductal homogeneous repartition in the cellular stroma as in the pericanalicular type of fibroadenoma.

190 HES ×10
Polypoid intracystic projections producing the so-called leaf pattern.

191 HES ×25
Intracystic projection: fibroblasts arranged perpendicularly to the axis (like veins of a leaf).

192 HES ×25
Cellularity is denser around epithelial clefts.

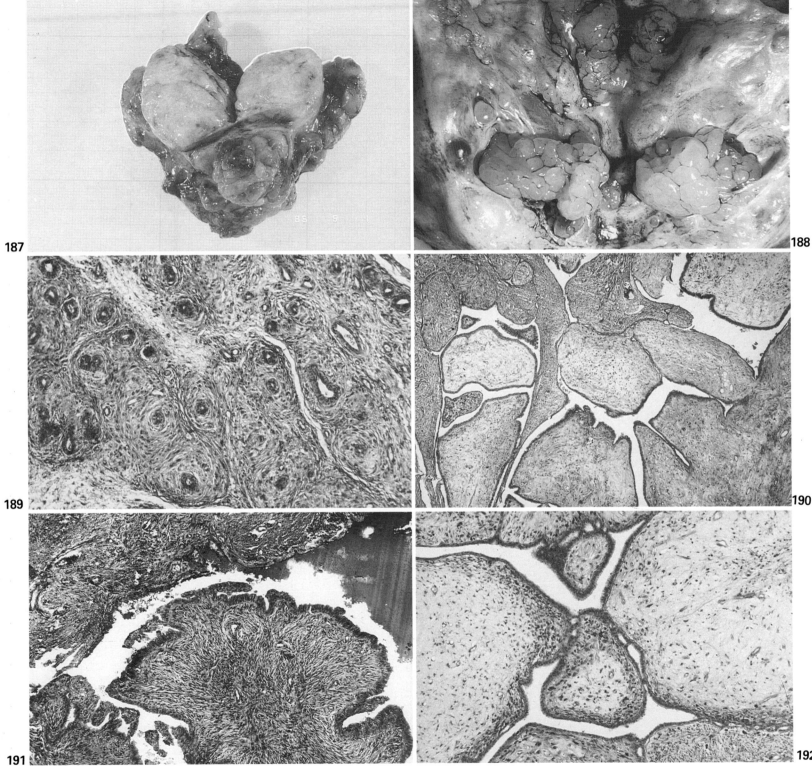

HISTOPROGNOSIS

The degree of aggressiveness cannot be predicted by only one histological factor but by the association of several:

- an infiltrating border;
- diffuse or localized disappearance of epithelical structures;
- high mitotic activity: probably the best malignancy index, but the rate assessed as indicator of malignancy varies according to studies (>3 or 10/10 HPF);
- moderate to marked cell atypia with possible malignant giant cells.
  But the absence of atypia does not indicate that the tumour is benign.

Three groups are constituted:

Tumour grade 1: benign
- 'pushing' border
- presence and homogeneous distribution of epithelial structures
- mitoses <3/10 HPF
- absent or discrete cell atypia.

Tumour grade 3: malignant
- 'infiltrating' border
- purely stromal nodules
- mitoses >10/10 HPF
- marked nuclear atypia.

Tumour grade 2: borderline malignant
  with one or two pejorative factors. This group has an unpredictable evolutive potential.

Phyllodes tumour grade 1

193 HES ×5
'Pushing' margin, hyalinized stroma.

194 HES ×64
Hypercellular stroma with regular fibroblasts.

Phyllodes tumour grade 2

195 HES ×25 ⎱
196 HES ×160 ⎰
Rare epithelial structures. The stroma is mucoid and not very cellular. Bizarre giant cells with hyperchromatic and multiple nuclei are scattered throughout the stroma.

　　However, the occurrence of bizarre giant cells in an otherwise benign appearing stroma does not constitute a sign of malignancy.

Phyllode grade 3

In decreasing frequency, the malignant stromal component presents as fibrosarcoma, liposarcoma, chondrosarcoma, osteosarcoma or rhabdomyosarcoma. Sometimes, the sarcoma is totally anaplastic.

197 HES ×64
Spindle-shaped cells with pleomorphic nuclei.

198 HES ×64
Areas of osteoid deposition within the sarcomatous stroma.

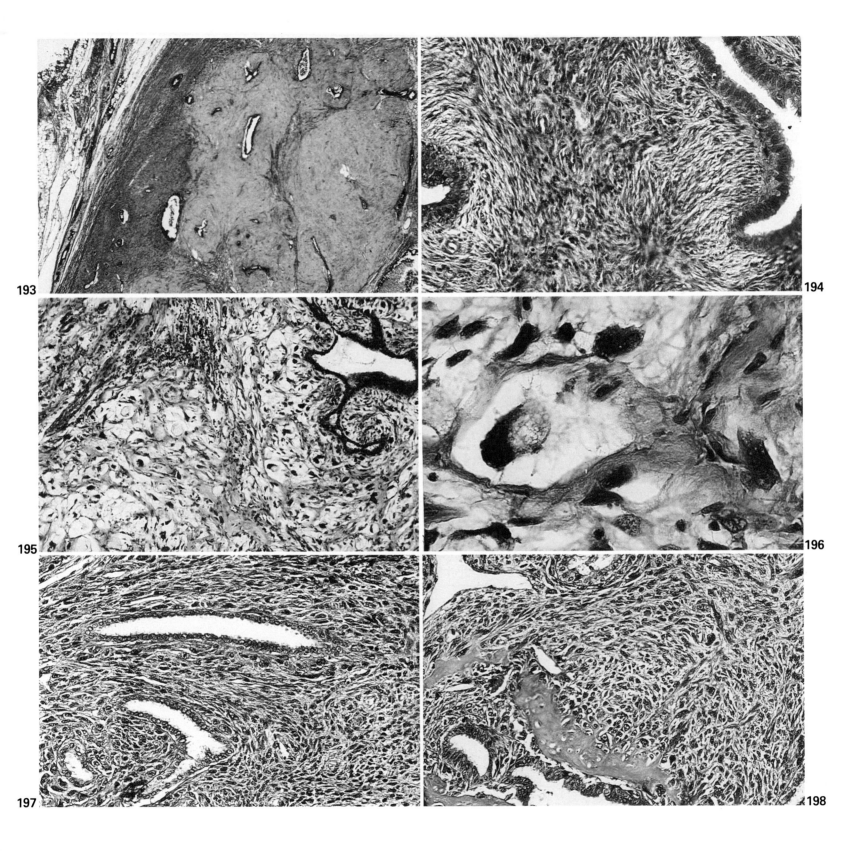

199 HES ×64
200 HES ×160
Grade 3: liposarcomatous differentiation.

201 HES ×25
202 HES ×64
Grade 3: liposarcomatous differentiation.

203 HES ×64
204 HES ×160
Grade 3: anaplastic area with malignant giant cells and abnormal mitoses.

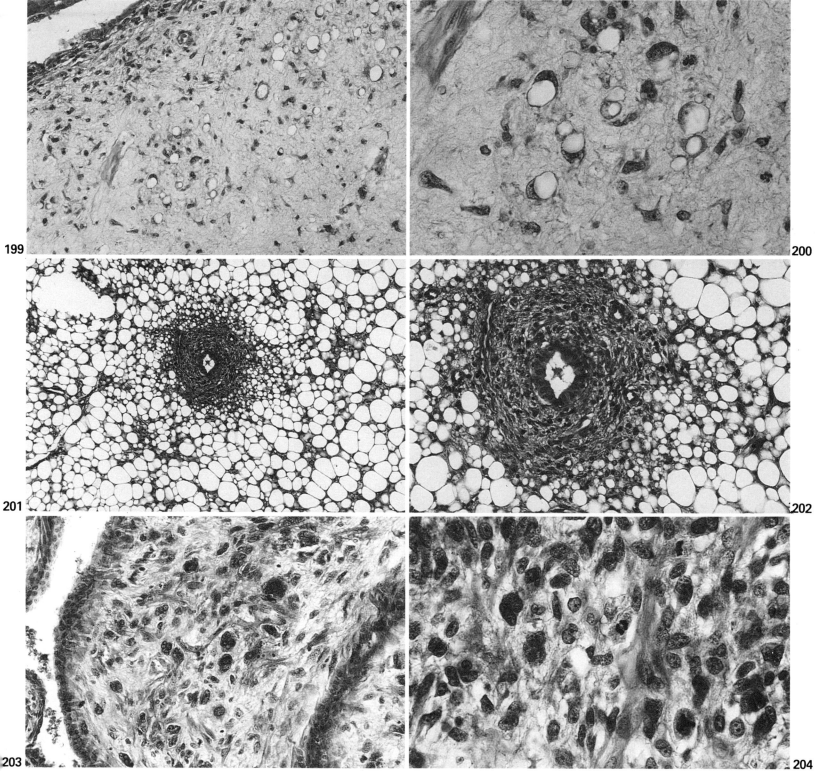

5.3 CARCINOSARCOMA

Definition

Tumour constituted by collision of two distinct malignant proliferations, a carcinomatous one originating from epithelial elements, and a sarcomatous one from stromal elements.

Therefore, true carcinosarcomas (in the histogenetic sense of the term) probably develop only from phyllodes tumours which have both an epithelial and a mesenchymal component.

Sarcomatous appearances in some carcinomas are currently considered as metaplastic (see metaplastic carcinomas Chapter 7, page 190).

Here is an example of carcinosarcoma in a patient presenting numerous bilateral fibroadenomas quiescent for years.

205 Mammography
Rapidly growing tumour with several calcified fibroadenomas.

206 Macroscopy
Solid, partially lobulated tumour.

207 HES ×5
Remnants of phyllodes tumour near a carcinomatous area.

208 HES ×25
Area of invasive carcinoma.

209 HES ×64
Carcinomatous area with 'cart-wheel' pattern.

210 HES ×64
Fibrosarcomatous area.

References
Chap. 5 – Fibroepithelial tumours

FIBROADENOMA

Ashikari, R. *et al.* (1971) Fibroadenomas in the breast of juveniles. *Surg. Gynecol. Obstet.*, **132**, 259.

Eusebi, V. *et al.* (1980) Lobular endocrine neoplasia in fibroadenoma of the breast. *Histopathology*, **4**, 413.

Fekete, P. *et al.* (1987) Fibroadenomas with stromal cellularity. *Arch. Pathol. Lab. Med.*, **111**, 427.

Fondo, E.Y. *et al.* (1979) The problem of carcinoma developing in a fibroadenoma. *Cancer*, **43**, 563.

Hertel, B.F. *et al.* (1976) Breast adenomas. *Cancer*, **37**, 2891.

Lacombe, M.J. *et al.* (1986) Fibroadénomes du sein avec hyperplasie épithéliale à cellules claires. *Ann. Pathol.*, **6**, 37.

Mies, C. and Rosen, P.P. (1987) Juvenile fibroadenoma with atypical epithelial hyperplasia. *Am. J. Surg. Pathol.*, **11**, 184.

Moross, T. *et al.* (1983) Tubular adenoma of breast. *Arch. Pathol. Lab. Med.*, **107**, 84.

Ozello, L. *et al.* (1985) The management of patients with carcinomas in fibroadenomatous tumours of the breast. *Surg. Gynecol. Obstet.*, **16**, 99.

Pike, A.M. *et al.* (1985) Juvenile (cellular) adenofibromas. *Am. J. Surg. Pathol.*, **9**, 730.

Sheth, M.T. *et al.* (1976) Pleomorphic adenoma (mixed tumour) of human female breast. *Cancer*, **41**, 659.

PHYLLODES TUMOUR

Austin, R.M. and Dupree, W.B. (1986) Liposarcoma of the breast. *Hum. Pathol.*, **17**, 906.

Briggs, R.M. *et al.* (1983) Cystosarcoma phyllodes in adolescent female patients. *Am. J. Surg.*, **146**, 172.

Lindquist, K.D. *et al.* (1982) Recurrent and metastatic cystosarcoma phyllodes. *Am. J. Surg.*, **144**, 341.

Norris, H.J. *et al.* (1967) Relationship of histologic features to behaviour of cystosarcoma phyllodes. *Cancer*, **20**, 2090.

Pietruszka, M. *et al.* (1978) Cystosarcoma phyllodes. *Cancer*, **41**, 1974.

Rosenfeld, J.C. *et al.* (1981) Cystosarcoma phyllodes. *Cancer Clin. Trials*, **4**, 187.

Treves, N. *et al.* (1951) Cystosarcoma phyllodes of the breast. *Cancer*, **4**, 1286.

CARCINOSARCOMA

Harris, M. *et al.* (1974) Carcinosarcoma of the breast. *J. Pathol.*, **112**, 99.

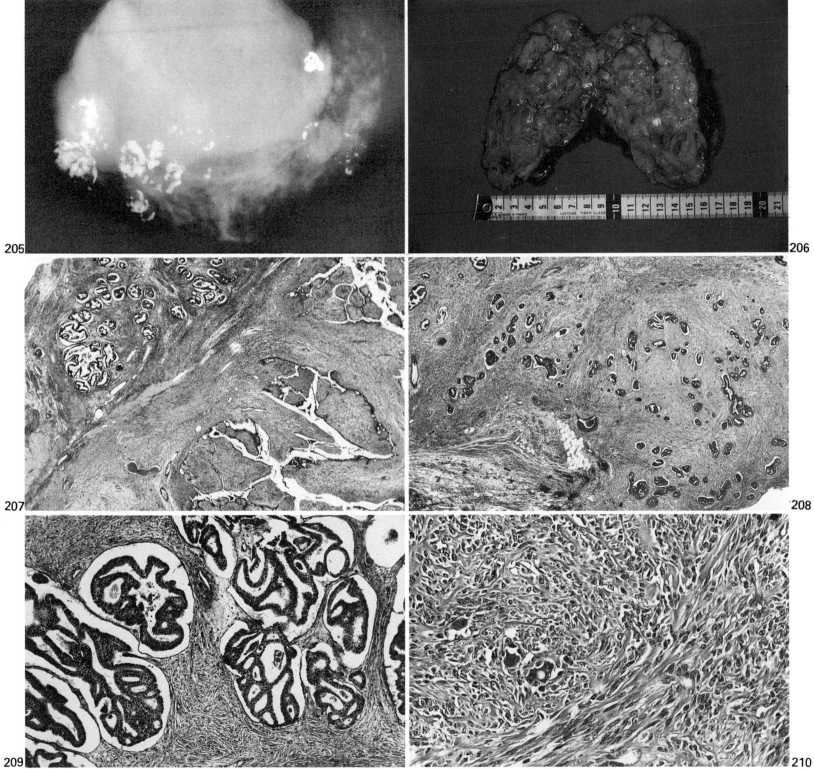

205

206

207

208

209

210

6

Miscellaneous benign entities

In this chapter, various lesions of low incidence (tumoural or not) are grouped: it is not an exhaustive list of all rare benign mammary lesions, but the author's personal choice.

6.1 Hemangioma
6.2 Fibromatosis
6.3 Hamartoma
6.4 Granulomatous mastitis
6.5 Spontaneous breast infarction
6.6 Fat necrosis
6.7 Fibrous disease of the breast
6.8 Granular cell tumour
6.9 Gynecomastia

6.1 HEMANGIOMA

Definition

Benign vascular lesion developed within the mammary gland.

1. *Microscopic perilobular hemangioma* composed of small capillary-sized blood vessels involving lobular stroma.
   (i) incidental finding in mammary tissue specimens (1%) or autopsies (11%),
   (ii) solitary or multiple, always benign.

2. *Macroscopic vascular tumour:* small-sized tumour which may be palpable but does not fill the criteria for angiosarcoma. Usually, the tumour is smaller than 2cm in its greatest diameter; there are no anastomosing vascular channels, atypical nuclei, endothelial papillary hyperplasia, spindle-cell component, mitoses or necrosis.

- **To distinguish a parenchymal from a subcutaneous hemangioma. The first one is very rare and often corresponds to a misdiagnosed angiosarcoma, when it gives a palpable tumour.**
- **Remember that some angiosarcomas can look histologically benign.**

---

211 HES ×25
Perilobular hemangioma: capillary-sized vessels intermingled with lobular epithelial structures.

212–214
Example of a 75-year-old woman presenting a palpable breast mass. The breast is atrophic and in adipose involution. Therefore it is difficult to determine the subcutaneous or intra-parenchymal site of the tumour.

212 Macroscopy
1.5cm dark tumour with ill-defined contours in an adipose tissue.

213 HES ×1
The mount section shows an angioma extending into fat.

214 HES ×10
Large cavernous blood vessels, independent of each other, without features of angiosarcoma.

6.2 FIBROMATOSIS

Synonym

Extra-abdominal desmoid.

Definition

Well-differentiated fibroblastic proliferation with abundant interstitial collagen, histologically benign, locally invasive and recurrent, giving no metastasis.

- **Primary mammary site very rare.**
- **Clinical and radiological signs are consistent with a carcinoma.**
- **Pathological features are typical (a little more difficult on frozen sections) and should not lead to error.**
- **Local excision must be wide to avoid recurrences which appear less frequently than in other sites.**

---

215 HES ×1
A whole mount section shows an infiltrating border with stellate extensions into the surrounding fat.

216 HES ×25
Typical pathological features: proliferation of regular fibroblasts with abundant interstitial collagen and numerous small vessels. The proliferation tends to grow around small ducts without destroying them.

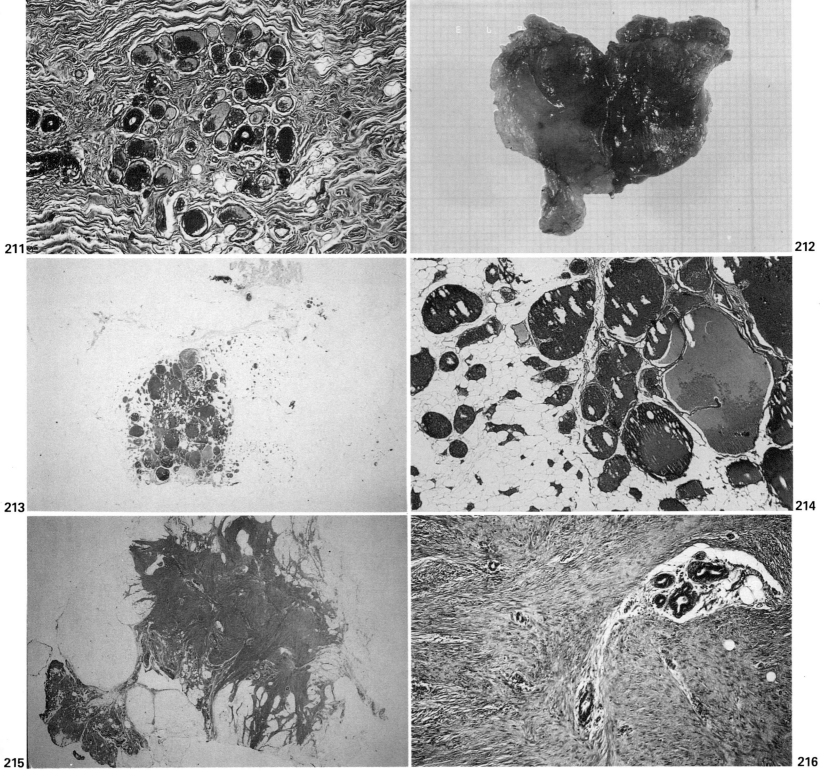

211

212

213

214

215

216

6.3 BREAST HAMARTOMA

Synonyms

Adenolipoma, fibroadenolipoma, mastoma, muscular or myoid hamartoma, post-lactational breast tumour.

Definition

Well-circumscribed tumour-like breast lesion, consisting of a mixture of normal breast tissue components ('a breast within the breast').

The clinical and pathological features depend on the proportion of these various elements:

- resembling a lipoma: if the adipose tissue is predominant; the tumour is hardly palpable, radiolucent.
- resembling a fibroadenoma: if the fibrous tissue and epithelial structures predominate; the tumour is firm and palpable, with mammographic mixed density.

In all cases, the tumour is totally circumscribed and separated from the adjacent breast tissue.

HAMARTOMA WITH A PREDOMINANCE OF FAT

217 Mammography
Voluminous radiolucent tumour surrounded by a capsule.

218 Macroscopy
The cut surface is soft, yellow and glistening (lipoma-like).

219 HES ×25
Periphery of the tumour with the capsule.

220 HES ×64
Smooth muscle differentiation near the capsule.

HAMARTOMA WITH AN EPITHELIAL PREDOMINANCE

221 HES ×1
A whole mount section shows an encapsulated lesion with numerous lobular groupings within adipose tissue.

222 HES ×25
Some lobules scattered in the adipose tissue.

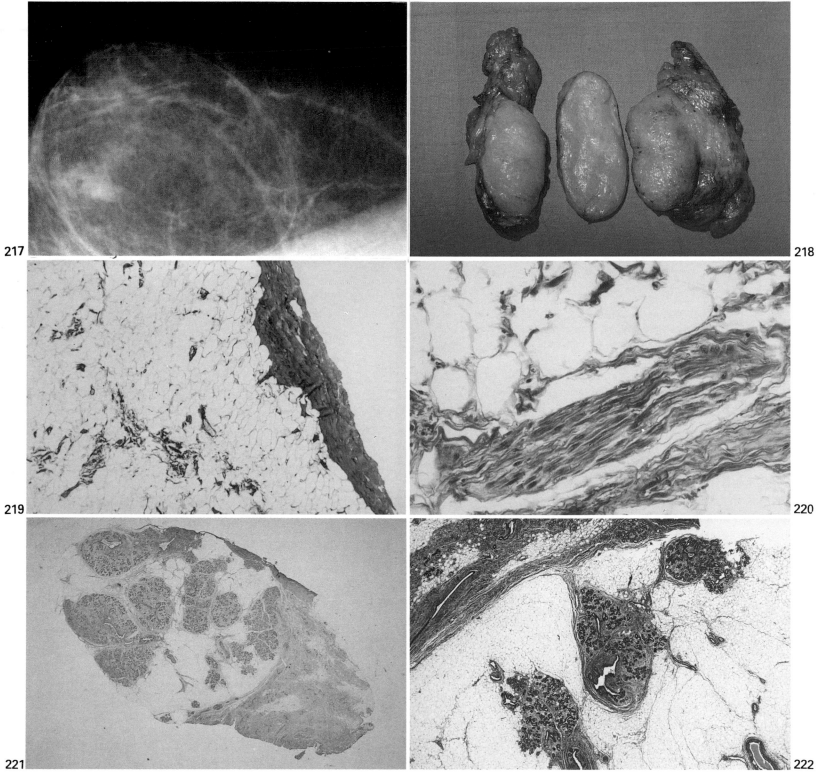

217

218

219

220

221

222

6.4 GRANULOMATOUS MASTITIS

Definition

Inflammatory lesion characterized by epithelioid and giant cell granulomas and abscesses confined to the lobules. All patients are young women of child-bearing age, presenting 1 to 5 years after their last delivery.

Etiology is unknown, the infectious origin has never been proved. An auto-immune process might be responsible for the development of the lesion.

Evolution: chronic and recurrent. In case of failure of classical treatment (antibiotics and non-steroidal anti-inflammatory drugs), it can be cured by corticoids.

> This lesion can mimic a carcinoma, clinically (hard and undefined nodule sometimes with skin retraction), radiologically (opacity with undefined contours and variable density).

Must be distinguished from other mastitis, tuberculosis, sarcoidosis and particularly plasma cell mastitis (in granulomatous mastitis, lobular site and absence of duct ectasia).

223 Mount section

224 HES ×10
Typical localization of inflammation within lobules.

225 HES ×64
Sarcoid reaction with epithelioid and giant cells (must be distinguished from a true sarcoidosis usually systemic and rare in mammary localization).

226 HES ×25
Granuloma destroying the lobule with micro-abscess.

6.5 SPONTANEOUS BREAST INFARCTION

Definition

Well-circumscribed tumour-like area of coagulative type necrosis of the mammary tissue. This lesion occurs in late pregnancy or early postpartum. Such an infarction can also occur in a fibroadenoma or an intraductal papilloma (may be associated with pregnancy and lactation).

Features
- Palpable lesion
- No mammographic signs
- Macroscopy: well-circumscribed firm nodule
- Microscopy: the nodule consists of a central area of necrosis with shadow glandular structures and a peripheral zone of granulation tissue.

> In some cases, the lesion can clinically mimic a carcinoma.

Pathogenesis

It still remains obscure: vascular insufficiency due to increased metabolism imposed by pregnancy or lactation?

227 HES ×1
The mount section shows a well-circumscribed nodule; the centre is occupied by necrosis and the periphery by distorted lobules and granulation tissue.

228 HES ×25
Coagulative type necrosis with shadow lobules.

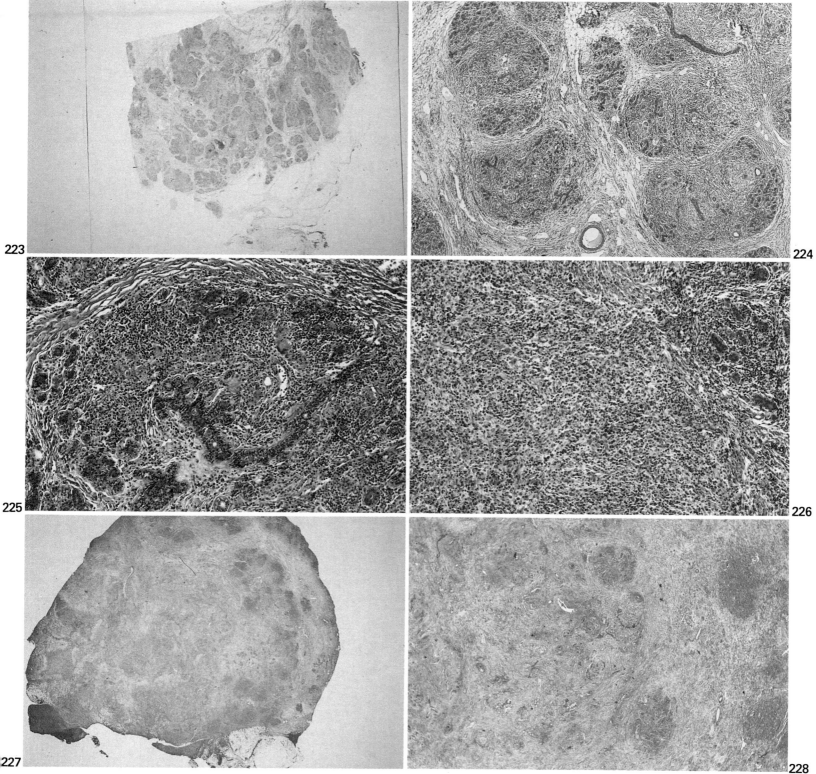

6.6 FAT NECROSIS

Definition

Tumour-like lesion due to traumatic destruction of adipose tissue (severe traumatism).

This lesion presents with two progressive stages:

> - *An early stage* (some days after injury). Diagnosis is easy because of a history of trauma and the contrast between the absence of radiological signs and the presence of a palpable nodule.
> - *A late stage* (some weeks or months or years after injury). The story of trauma is often forgotten and there is a tumour simulating a cancer.

EARLY STAGE: destruction of adipocytes, macrophagic reaction

229 Macroscopy
Soft, yellow usually localized area in the superficial subcutaneous tissue.

230 HES ×64
Destroyed adipocytes liberate lipids constituting vacuoles surrounded by giant cells and foamy histiocytes.

LATE STAGE: fibrous scar

231 Mammography
Carcinoma-like aspect with disorganization of trabeculae and skin thickening.

232 Mammography
Sclerosis and radiolucent cyst, the appearance of which is typical of an oil cyst.

233 HES ×64
Inflammation with interstitial discrete fibrosis.

234 HES ×25
Marked fibrosis with disappearance of granuloma and cyst formation.

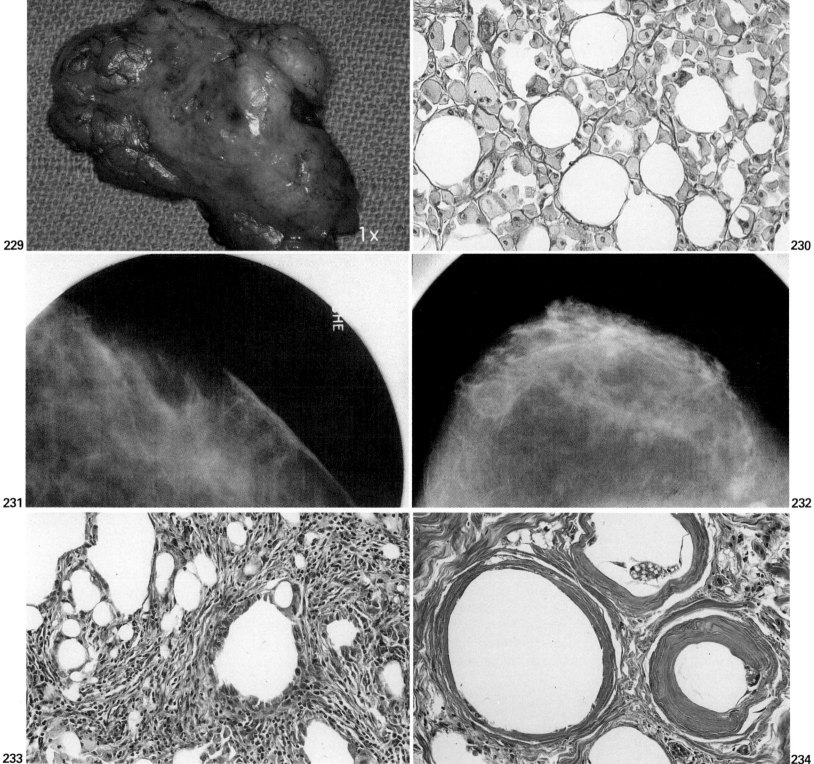

229

230

231

232

233

234

6.7 FIBROUS DISEASE OF THE BREAST

Synonyms

Focal fibrous disease, fibrous mastopathy, chronic indurative mastitis, fibrous dysplasia.

Definition

Localized area of fibrosis that leads to the progressive and sometimes complete disappearance of TDLU.

Features

- rare disease developing during age of fertility;
- palpable tumour; at mammography, opacity with irregular outline, sometimes simulating a carcinoma;
- histologically: typical features (Figures 235–239).

Genesis

It is debatable whether this is a true disease entity or only a variant of normal mammary involution. The presence of this lesion in young women argues in favour of the first hypothesis. The origin remains obscure: perhaps inflammatory or vascular.

235 HES ×1
A mount section shows a circumscribed fibrous nodule within a mammary parenchyma. The fibrosis is acellular, punctuated with rare lobules or ducts that are gradually disappearing.

236 HES ×64
A lobule with discrete lymphocytic infiltration and early centrolobular fibrosis.

237 HES ×64
Marked lymphocytic infiltrate with partial lobular destruction.

238 HES ×64
Lymphocytic infiltrate without any epithelial remnant.

239 HES ×25
Fibrosis with destruction of lobular epithelial structures.

6.8 GRANULAR CELL TUMOUR

Synonym

Myoblastoma, Abrikossoff's tumour.

Tumour composed of large cells with granular cytoplasm stained with S100 protein; its histogenesis is controversial (neurogenic origin currently admitted). This benign tumour is found anywhere in the body and its mammary localization must be mentioned only because it may simulate a carcinoma, clinically (very firm consistency, skin retraction), mammographically (dense, ill-circumscribed nodule) and pathologically (mistaken for a carcinoma, on frozen sections).

240 HES ×64
Tumour cells with small nuclei and large granular cytoplasm, surrounding small ducts.

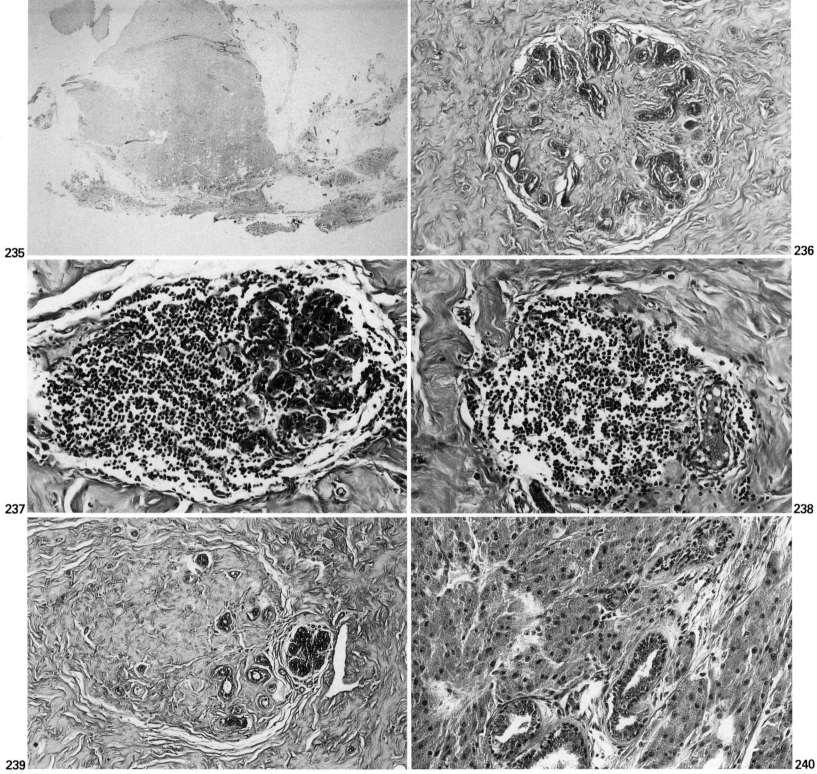

6.9 GYNECOMASTIA

Definition

Enlargement of the male breast.

High frequency (up to 40% in a series of autopsies). Excision is performed (except for aesthetic purposes) only if there is suspicion of carcinoma (asymmetric and irregular hypertrophy).

Gynecomastia is not a precancerous lesion (except if associated with a Klinefelter's syndrome).

Histology

There are three types (Williams, 1963):
1. florid: oestrogen therapy gives this aspect;
2. quiescent: the most common;
3. dissociated aspect: the rarest.

- The histological types are not progressive stages of the lesion.
- The element which appears predominant in the lesion is the destruction of elastic tissue and changes of connective tissue.

---

241 HES ×5
242 HES ×25

Gynecomastia type I: duct hyperplasia and epithelial hyperplasia with pseudopapillary tufts. A loose oedematous stroma with rare collagen fibres surrounds the ducts.

243 HES ×25
244 HES ×25

Gynecomastia type II: ducts surrounded by a dense collagen, without epithelial hyperplasia.

245 HES ×25
246 HES ×64

Gynecomastia type III: ductal epithelial hyperplasia but dense collagen. Here, the hyperplasia might be alarming because of a pseudocribriform pattern, but there is never cellular polarity found in DCIS bridges.

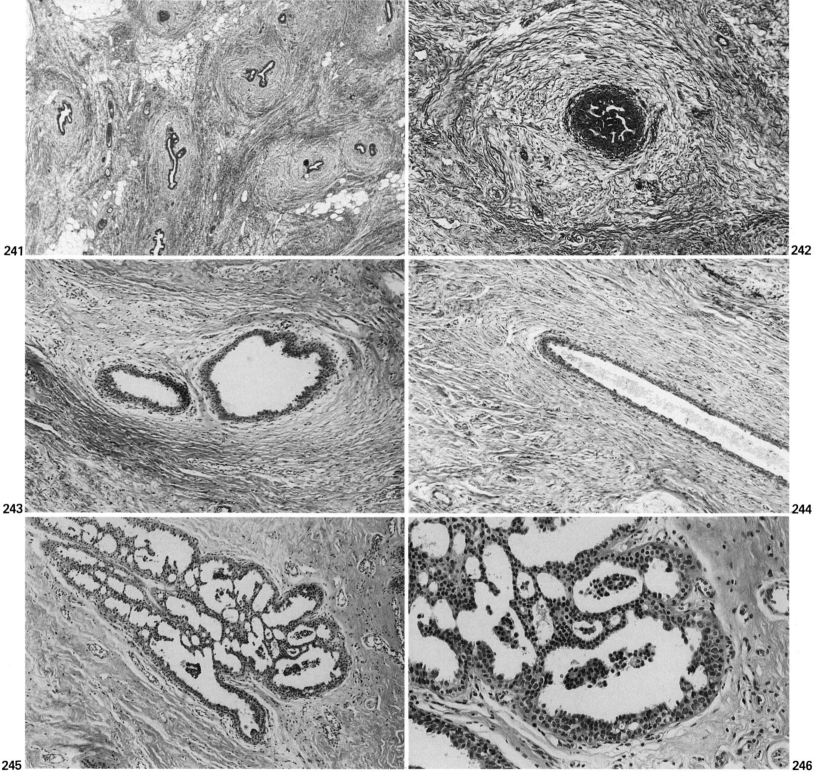

241

242

243

244

245

246

References
Chap. 6 – Miscellaneous Benign Lesions

HEMANGIOMA

Josefczyk, M.A. *et al.* (1985) Vascular tumors of the breast. II. Perilobular hemangiomas and hemangiomas. *Am. J. Surg.*, **9**, 491.

Lesueur, G.C. *et al.* (1983) Incidence of perilobular hemangioma in the female breast. *Arch. Pathol. Lab. Med.*, **107**, 308.

Rosen, P.P. *et al.* (1985) Vascular tumors of the breast. III. Angiomatosis. *Am. J. Surg. Pathol.*, **9**, 652. IV. Venous hemangiomas. *Am. J. Surg. Pathol.*, **9**, 649. V. Non-parenchymal hemangiomas of mammary subcutaneous tissue. *Am. J. Surg. Pathol.*, **9**, 723.

FIBROMATOSIS

Enzinger, F.M. and Weiss, S.W. (1983) Soft tissue tumors. Saint-Louis, C. V. Mosby, 53–62.

Gad, A. *et al.* (1983–1984) Fibromatose du sein: une lésion qui simule un cancer. *Int. J. Mammary Pathol. Senologia*, **2**, 197.

Gump, F.E. *et al.* (1981) Fibromatosis of the breast. *Surg. Gynecol. Obstet.*, **153**, 57.

Wargotz, E.S. *et al.* (1987) Fibromatosis of the breast. *Am. J. Surg. Pathol.*, **11**, 38.

HAMARTOMA

Daroca, P.J. *et al.* (1985) Myoid hamartomas of the breast. *Hum. Pathol.*, **16**, 212.

Goussot *et al.* (1983) Hamartomes mammaires. *Arch. Anat. Cytol. Pathol.*, **31**, 351.

Hessler, C. *et al.* (1978) Hamartoma of the breast. *Radiology*, **126**, 95.

Linell, F. *et al.* (1979) Breast hamartomas. *Virchows Arch.* (Pathol. Anat.), **383**, 253.

GRANULOMATOUS MASTITIS

Hertogh, D.A. *et al.* (1980) Prednisone management of granulomatous mastitis. *N. Engl. J. Med.*, **303**, 799.

Kessler, E. *et al.* (1972) Granulomatous mastitis. *Am. J. Clin. Pathol.*, **58**, 642.

Ross, M.J. *et al.* (1985) Sarcoidosis of the breast. *Hum. Pathol.*, **16**, 185.

Smadja, A. *et al.* (1977) La mastite granulomateuse (7 cas). *Gynécologie*, **28**, 209.

SPONTANEOUS BREAST INFARCTION

Jimenez, J.F. *et al.* (1986) Spontaneous breast infarction associated with pregnancy presenting as a palpable mass. *J. Surg. Oncol.*, **32**, 174.

Lucey, J.L. (1975) Spontaneous infarction of the breast. *J. Clin. Pathol.*, **28**, 937.

FAT NECROSIS

Adair, F.E. *et al.* (1947) Fat necrosis of the female breast; report of 110 cases. *Am. J. Surg.*, **74**, 117.

Bassett, L.W. *et al.* (1978) Mammographic spectrum of traumatic fat necrosis: the fallibility of 'pathognomonic signs of carcinoma'. *A.J.R.*, **130**, 119.

FIBROUS DISEASE OF THE BREAST

Hermann, G. *et al.* (1983) Focal fibrous disease of the breast. *A.J.R.*, **140**, 1245.

Rivera-Pomar, J.M. *et al.* (1980) Focal fibrous disease of breast. *Virchows Arch.* (Pathol. Anat.) **386**, 59.

GRANULOMA CELL TUMOUR

Bassett, L.W. *et al.* (1979) Myoblastoma of the breast. *A.J.R.*, **132**, 122.

Ingram, D.L. *et al.* (1984) Granular cell tumors of the breast. *Arch. Pathol. Lab. Med.*, **108**, 897.

Willen, R. *et al.* (1984) Granular cell tumour of the mammary gland simulating malignancy. *Virchows Arch.* (Pathol. Anat.), **403**, 391.

Zemoura, L. *et al.* (1984) Myoblastomes granuleux du sein. *Ann. Pathol.*, **4**, 151.

GYNECOMASTIA

Carlson, H.E. (1980) Gynaecomastia, *N. Engl. J. Med.*, **303**, 795.

Pages, A. *et al.* (1984) Contribution à l'étude des gynécomasties (122 cas). *Ann Pathol.*, **4**, 137.

Williams, M.J. (1963) Gynecomastia: its incidence, recognition and host characterization in 447 autopsy cases. *Am. J. Med.*, **34**, 103.

7

Carcinomas

The histological type of cancer is an important element in assisting in the establishment of prognosis and treatment. The multitude of proposed classifications does not make the comparison of results easier. In 1981, a group of WHO experts seeking a uniform terminology proposed an international classification which will serve as a basis for our study.

The definitions of the various histological types of carcinoma found in this atlas were taken from this publication.

Carcinomas represent 98% of malignant breast tumours and are classified as follows, according to WHO.

7.1 NON INVASIVE CARCINOMA

Lobular carcinoma in situ
Ductal carcinoma in situ

7.2 INVASIVE CARCINOMA

Invasive ductal carcinoma
Invasive ductal carcinoma with a predominant intraductal component
Invasive lobular carcinoma
Mucinous carcinoma
Medullary carcinoma
Papillary carcinoma
Tubular carcinoma
Adenoid cystic carcinoma
Apocrine carcinoma
Carcinoma with metaplasia
Carcinoma with spindle-cell metaplasia
Carcinoma with squamous metaplasia
Other invasive carcinomas

7.3 PAGET'S DISEASE OF THE NIPPLE

The site of origin of carcinomas has long been discussed. Wellings (1975) has shown that most of the carcinomas (lobular and ductal) start in the TDLU. Currently, most of the authors agree with this view. Thus the topographic criterion is no longer useful to distinguish between the lobular or ductal nature of a carcinoma.

7.4 COMBINATIONS OF HISTOLOGICAL TYPES IN THE SAME TUMOUR MASS

7.1 NON INVASIVE CARCINOMAS

LOBULAR CARCINOMA IN SITU (LCIS)

Synonym

Lobular neoplasia (however, this term includes atypical lobular hyperplasia; see page 82).

Definition

A carcinoma involving the intralobular ductules which are obliterated and distended by loosely aggregated cells without stromal invasion. The tumour cells may extend into extralobular ducts (pagetoid spread) and may replace the ductal epithelium.'

Clinical features

- **Rare form (2.5% of carcinomas)**
- **Incidental finding**
- **Mean age 45 years, in premenopausal women**
- *Bilaterality* **30%**
- *Multicentricity* **50–70%**
- **Possible occurrence of invasive carcinoma (20%) after a long interval (10 to 25 years).**

Histological features

- In *lobules*: acini are distended and obliterated by rounded and regular cells; the cells contain target-like mucinous cytoplasmic vacuoles, more frequent in lobular carcinoma than in other types of carcinoma;
- In *ducts*: the 'pagetoid spread' (see Glossary, page 11) constitutes a feature more frequent in lobular carcinoma in situ but which is not pathognomonic and can also be seen in ductal carcinoma in situ.

Differential diagnosis

- appearance of lobular carcinoma in situ due to bad fixation,
- with atypical lobular hyperplasia (ALH),
- with ductal carcinoma in situ (DCIS).

INVOLVEMENT OF LOBULES

247 HES ×10
Normal lobule contrasting with neoplastic lobule in which all acini are distended and obliterated by tumour cells.

248 HES ×160
Acini obliterated by regular calls.

249 D-PAS ×400
Target-like mucinous cytoplasmic inclusions. These target-like inclusions though not specific are very characteristic of breast carcinomas and are particularly frequent in lobular carcinomas.

250 HES ×400
Target-like cytoplasmic vacuole visible on routine stainings.

251 D-PAS ×25
252 D-PAS ×160
Lobule obliterated by LCIS, loss of cellular cohesiveness; intracytoplasmic mucinous vacuoles.

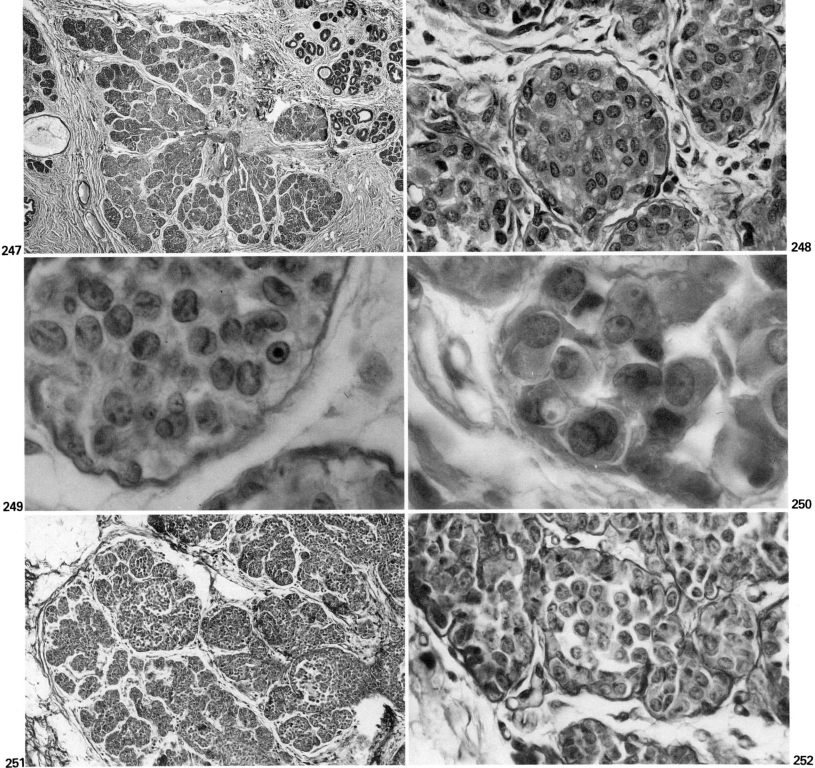

253   HES ×64 ⎫
254   HES ×160 ⎭
A lobule with a mixture of typical LCIS cells and closely packed hyperchromatic cells.

255   PAS ×160
LCIS: macro-acini.

256   HES ×160
Atypical cells in an otherwise typical LCIS.

257   HES ×64 ⎫
258   HES ×160 ⎭
LCIS with a mixture of typical areas and papillary structures.

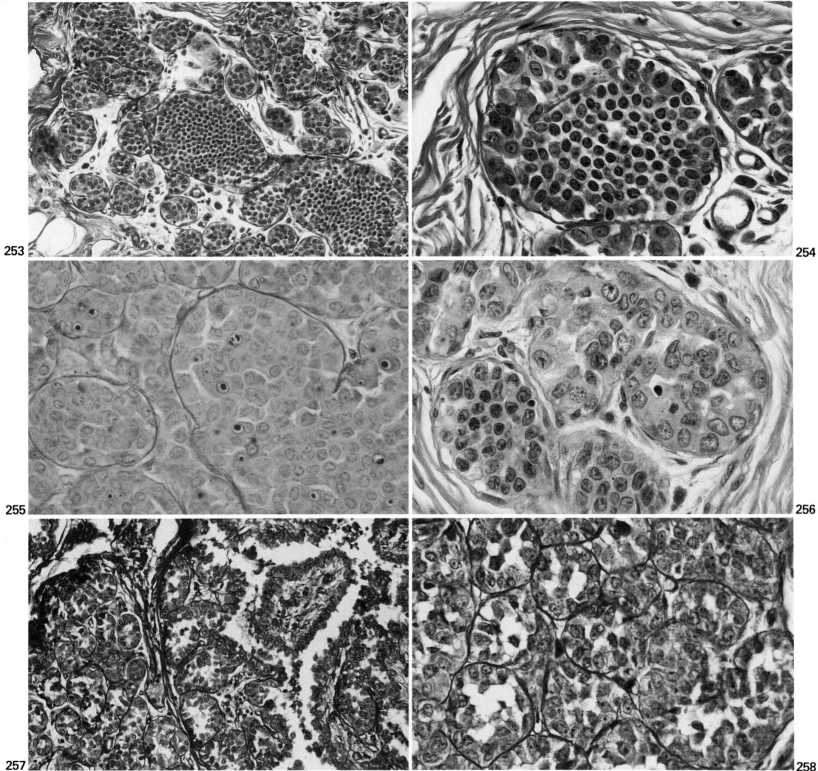

INVOLVEMENT OF DUCTS

The ducts can be affected by LCIS with a pagetoid-spread aspect more extensively than the lobules after menopause when the lobules become atrophic.

Within small ducts

259 HES ×25 ⎫
260 HES ×64 ⎭
The tumour cells spread beneath the epithelial cell layer and form a series of rounded projections into the breast stroma with a 'clover-leaf' pattern.
   The cells can also destroy the epithelial cell layer and obliterate the lumen of the duct.

Within larger ducts

261 HES ×160
The tumour cells are grouped between the basal membrane and the epithelial cell layer.

262 HES ×160
The tumour cells are sandwiched between the inner-epithelial cell layer and the outer-myoepithelial cell layer.

263 Cytok ×64
Neoplastic cells are strongly positive. Compare with a normal duct in which myoepithelial cells are negative.

264 S100 protein ×64
Neoplastic cells are negative. Compare with a normal duct in which myoepithelial cells are positive. A few myoepithelial cells persist between LCIS cells.

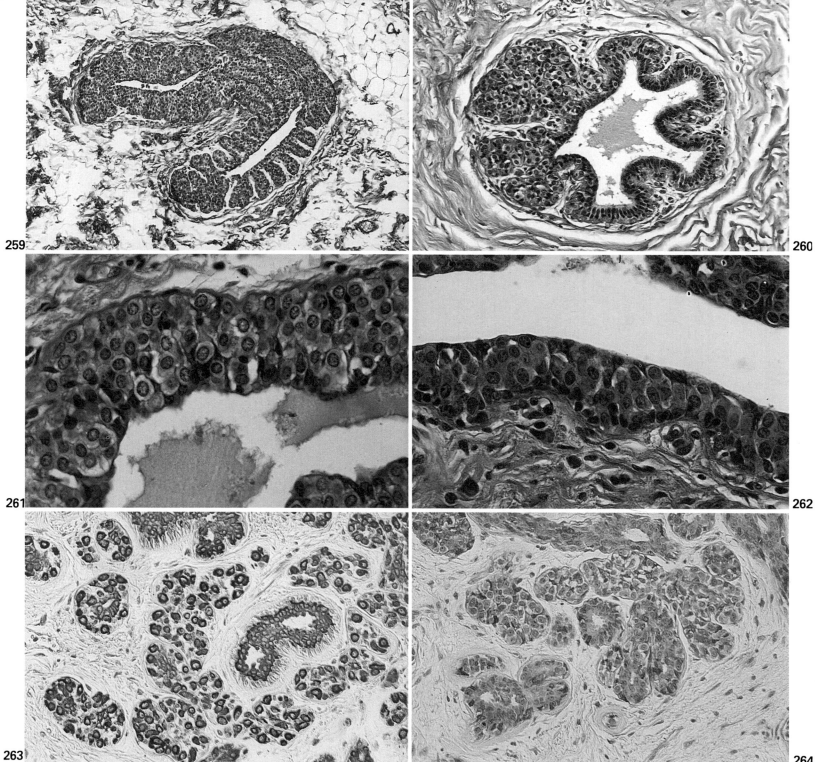

DIFFERENTIAL DIAGNOSIS
Misleading appearances of LCIS

Epithelial cells part from the acinus wall and seem to fill up lumina (because of insufficient or delayed fixation).

Atypical lobular hyperplasia

Atypical lobular hyperplasia (ALH) is defined according to WHO as a 'lesion which is similar to but quantitatively and qualitatively insufficient to support a diagnosis of lobular carcinoma in situ'. The persistence of luminal spaces, lack of marked ductular distension and the persistence of a myoepithelial cell layer help to distinguish atypical lobular hyperplasia from lobular carcinoma in situ.

The fragility of this distinction and the very subjective assessment from one observer to another must be underlined.

Haagensen (1978) groups atypical lobular hyperplasia and lobular carcinoma in situ under the name of 'lobular neoplasia'.

For others, atypical lobular hyperplasia and lobular carcinoma in situ are the two extremes of a lesional continuum but the risk factor of subsequent invasive carcinoma is probably higher for LCIS than for ALH.

265 HES ×64
266 HES ×160
Appearance of LCIS because of inadequately fixed material.

267 HES ×25
268 HES ×64
ALH: not very distended acini, visible lumina, cells not characteristic of LCIS.

269 PAS ×64
270 HES ×160
The partial invasion of the lobule by LCIS is possible and does not exclude this diagnosis, particularly when cells are typical of this carcinoma. However, many observers would classify this lesion as ALH.

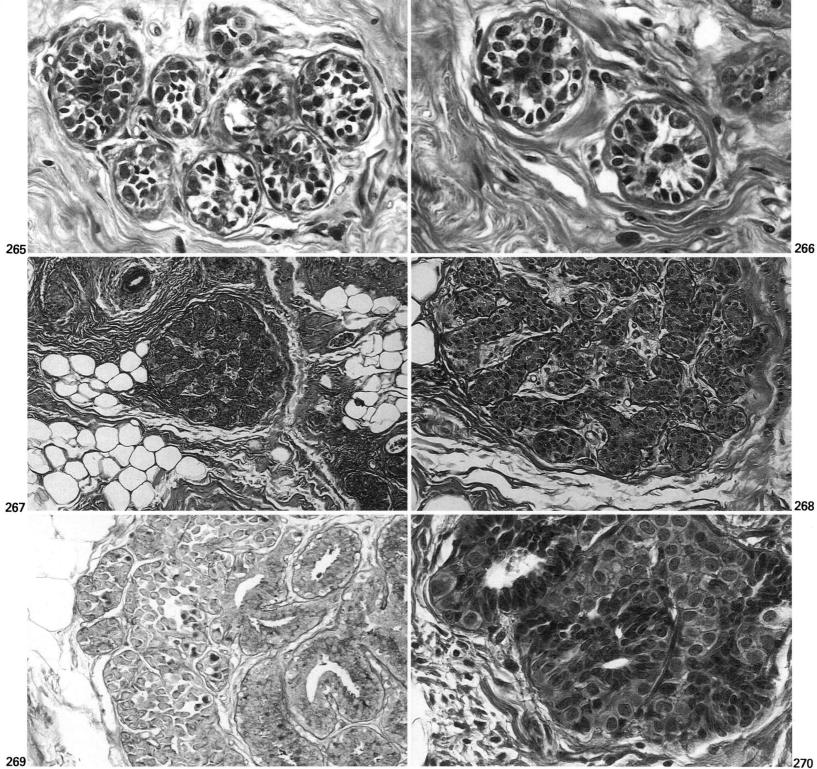

DIFFERENTIAL DIAGNOSIS
with ductal carcinoma in situ

This diagnosis is discussed in three conditions:

1. When ductal carcinoma in situ is localized within lobules, i.e. 'lobular cancerization'. The diagnosis of ductal carcinoma in situ is easy if cells are atypical but if cells are small and if there is an intraductal necrosis, the diagnosis between ductal carcinoma in situ and lobular carcinoma in situ is difficult;

2. When there are features of 'pagetoid spread'. The diagnosis of ductal carcinoma in situ is easy if cells are atypical, but if cells are small, the diagnosis between ductal carcinoma in situ and lobular carcinoma in situ is difficult or impossible;

3. When there is coexistence of lobular carcinoma in situ and ductal carcinoma in situ. This coexistence is not obvious if both processes are comprised of small cells.

Lobular cancerization

271   HES ×10 ⎫
272   HES ×64 ⎭
Here, the diagnosis of ductal carcinoma in situ is based on the following arguments:
- marked difference in size of acini,
- massive injection of the extralobular terminal duct with persistence of normal acini,
- presence of cribriform pattern.

273   HES ×25
Cells are of lobular type but central necrosis can lead one to suspect a comedo type ductal carcinoma in situ.
Note: when this feature is found in a lobular carcinoma in situ, an associated invasive lobular carcinoma must be suspected.

Pagetoid spread

274   HES ×160
The diagnosis of lobular carcinoma in situ is favoured in the presence of many mucinous intra-cytoplasmic vacuoles. But it is not a formal argument.

Coexistence of lobular carcinoma in situ and ductal carcinoma in situ

275   HES ×10 ⎫
276   HES ×64 ⎭
Coexistence of lobular carcinoma in situ and ductal carcinoma in situ in the same lobule. The architectural and cytologic features of both processes are clearly distinct.

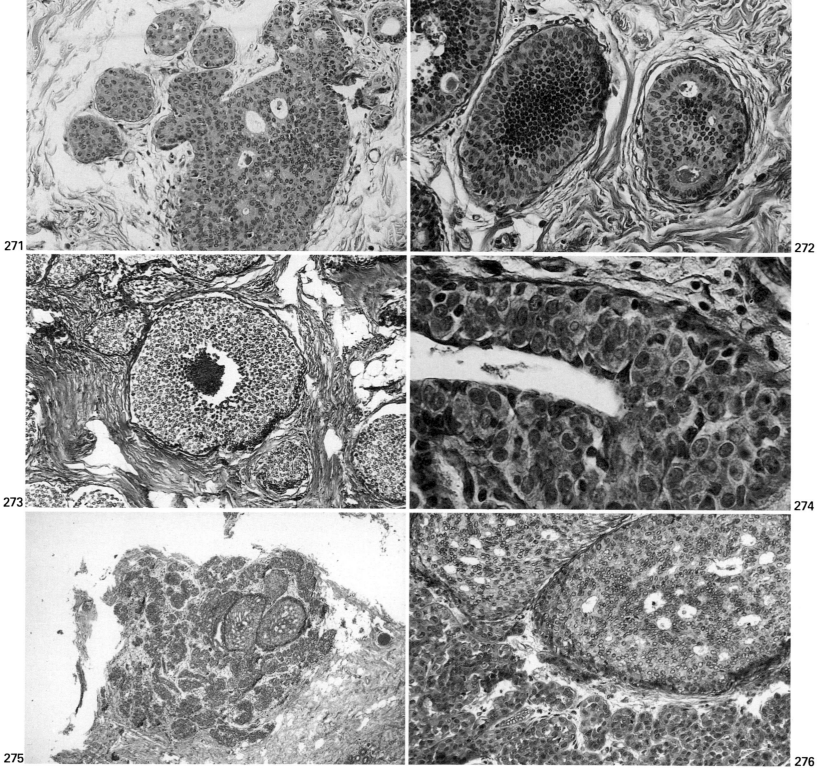

277 HES ×25 ⎱
278 HES ×64 ⎰
Coexistence of lobular carcinoma in situ and ductal carcinoma in situ: lobular carcinoma in situ cells go into the epithelium of ductal carcinoma in situ papillae.

279 HES ×64 ⎱
280 HES ×64 ⎰
Mixed growth pattern of both lobular carcinoma in situ and ductal carcinoma in situ but with similar cells. The diagnosis is difficult and uncertain between ductal carcinoma in situ only, or coexistence of lobular carcinoma in situ with ductal carcinoma in situ.

281 HES ×25 ⎱
282 HES ×64 ⎰
Presence within the same ducts of lobular carcinoma in situ and apocrine ductal carcinoma in situ. The latter shows glandular differentiation.

DUCTAL CARCINOMA IN SITU (DCIS)

Definition

'A carcinoma of mammary ducts which does not invade the surrounding stroma and is characterized by four growth patterns: solid, comedo, papillary and cribriform. Failure to identify stromal invasion simply means that it has not been demonstrated but does not rule it out.'

Terminology – Nosology (Figure 286)

Clinical features

- Rare form: 4% of carcinomas.
- Detection: tumour, bloody discharge, Paget's disease, microcalcifications.
- Mean age: 54 years.
- Bilaterality: 10%.
- Multicentricity: 30%.
- Recurrence: particularly after simple excision, as intraductal or invasive. The frequency varies according to the published series (10 to 70%). Further investigations are necessary to understand the natural history of DCIS.

Histological features

- Growth patterns: solid, comedo, cribriform, papillary, mixed, clinging (see pages 120 to 125).
- Cells: the largest number of atypical cells in the comedo type, frequency of round nuclei.
- Variants: intracystic, apocrine, mucinous, within duct ectasia (pages 134 to 137),
- Multicentricity (page 138–139):
  - intraductal spread and/or multiple foci *de novo*,
  - lobular cancerization and pagetoid spread.

Differential diagnosis

- with benign lesions: epitheliosis, blunt duct adenosis, atypical ductal hyperplasia,
- with other malignant lesions: lobular carcinoma in situ (page 116), microinvasive intraductal carcinoma, invasive ductal carcinoma, adenoid cystic carcinoma (page 188).

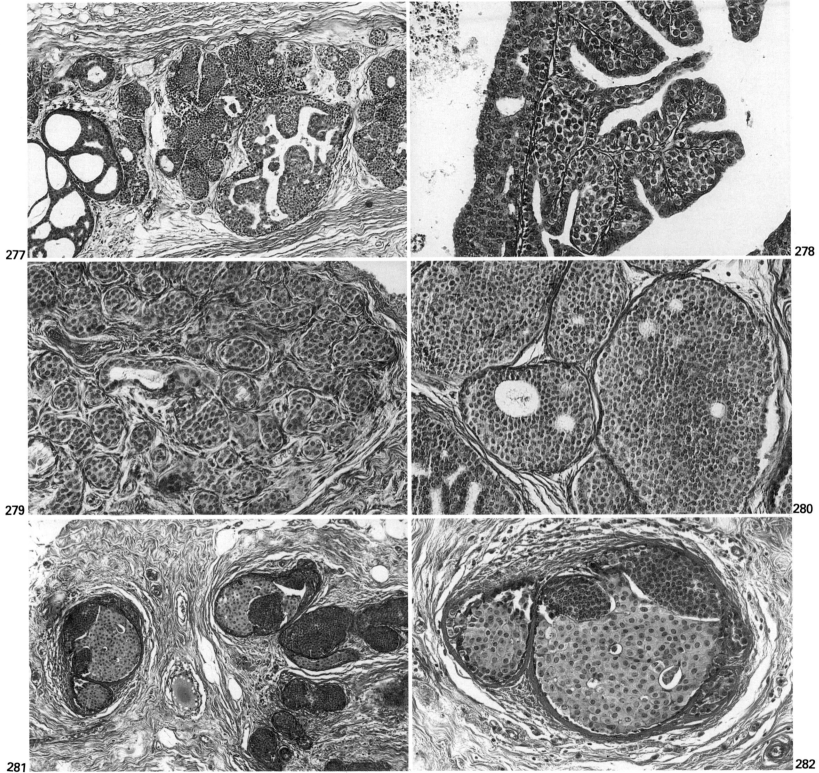

MAMMOGRAPHY

The image may be either a tumour mass with ill-defined or unsharp contours, or isolated micro-calcifications, characteristic by their number, arrangement, shape and grouping.

MACROSCOPY

The ductal carcinoma in situ may correspond to a tumour mass with irregular margins or to a firm, ill-individualized area of mammary tissue. It also may be totally invisible. A characteristic gross feature of ductal carcinoma in situ is the presence of comedones (so called due to the analogy with cutaneous comedones). They are small yellowish cylinders which spring up under the pressure. They histologically correspond to intraductal necrosis (see comedo type).

GROWTH PATTERNS

Note:
- On the one hand, the same term for a given pattern does not systematically correspond to the same histological aspects; thus, the papillary pattern may correspond only to true papillae with a fibrous stalk, or else to pseudopapillary epithelial projections without a fibrous stalk.
- On the other hand, a mixture of all patterns usually occurs, although any one may predominate.

Haagensen (1986) defines a carcinoma as intraductal 'only when 50% of the lesion has an intraductal format'. He refutes the term of 'noninvasive' carcinoma, considering that any carcinoma may invade somewhere but that this invasion may not be demonstrated by the pathologist through light microscopy.

283 Mammography
Clusters of irregular microcalcifications extending from the nipple towards the depth of the breast.

284 Mammography
One cluster of microcalcifications irregular in shape.

285 Macroscopy
Ill-defined tumour; pressure pushes out comedones.

286 Diagram of growth patterns in a few classifications.

287 HES ×25 ⎫
288 HES ×25 ⎭
Solid pattern: the ductal lumen is totally obliterated by the proliferation.

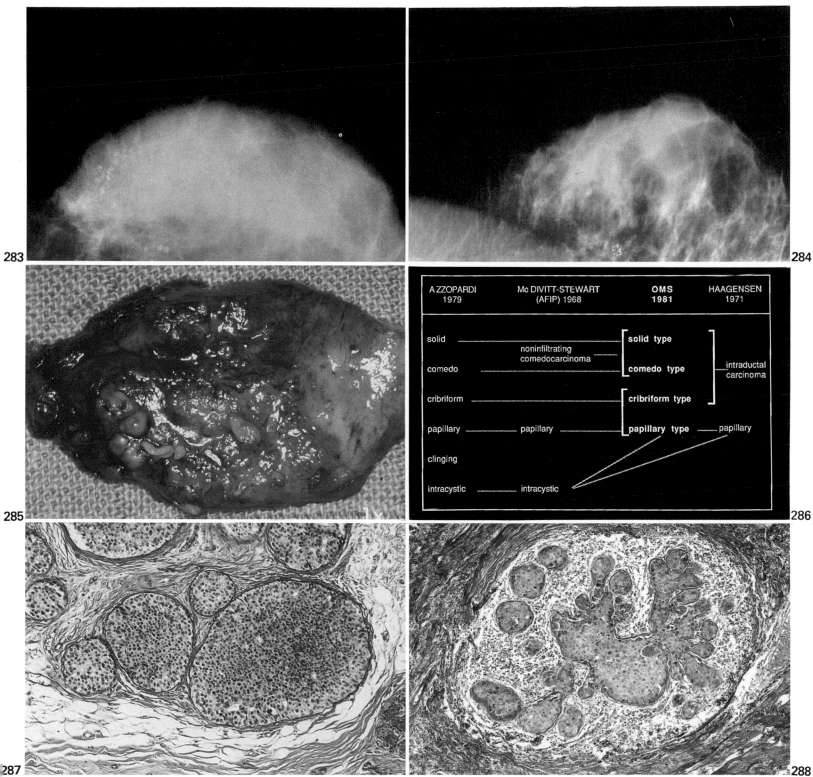

A ZZOPARDI 1979	Mc DIVITT-STEWART (AFIP) 1968	OMS 1981	HAAGENSEN 1971
solid		**solid type**	
	noninfiltrating comedocarcinoma		intraductal carcinoma
comedo		**comedo type**	
cribriform		**cribriform type**	
papillary	papillary	**papillary type**	papillary
clinging			
intracystic	intracystic		

289 HES ×25 ⎱
290 HES ×10 ⎰
Comedo type: central necrosis which may be total up to the basement membrane. This feature is considered as being more frequently associated with a microinvasive process.

291 HES ×10
Cribriform type: solid-tumour growth is interrupted by small round rigid holes around which columnar cells have a glandular polarity.

292 HES ×25
Papillary type: true papillae with a fibrous stalk.

293 HES ×160
A papilla covered with several epithelial layers but with one cell type; disappearance of the myoepithelial layer.

294 HES ×160
A papilla covered with one epithelial layer with disappearance of the myoepithelial layer and crowding of the epithelium.

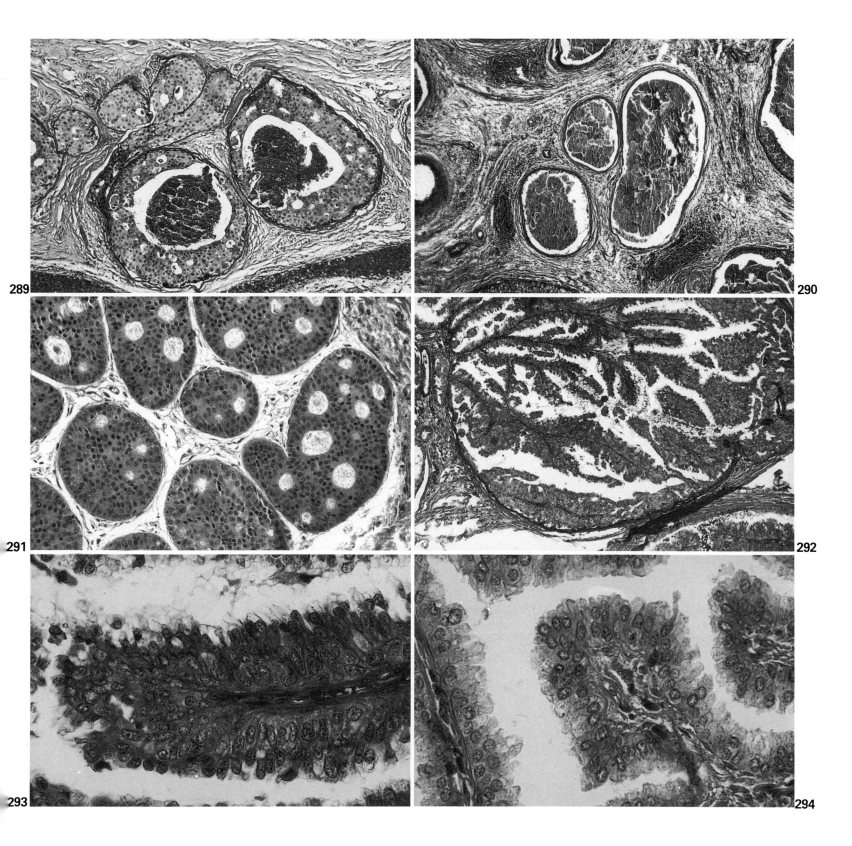

295 HES ×64
Papillary type: reticular pattern, long and thin epithelial projections without fibrous stalk that merge in the lumen and constitute a network.

296 HES ×25
Papillary type: finger-like pattern (McDivitt), i.e. thin and short epithelial projections without fibrous stalk.

297 HES ×25
298 HES ×64
Papillary type: daisy-like aggregates, small rounded epithelial tufts becoming free in the lumen. These tufts appear aciniform with peripheric arrangement of nuclei but without central lumen.

299 HES ×25
Papillary type: large circular spaces with the appearance of bridges or trabecular bars or 'radial spokes of a wheel'. Various names are found in the literature: 'bridge arch' pattern, 'lace-like' pattern, 'cart-wheel' pattern. This papillary type is classified according to the authors as either papillary or cribriform.

300 HES ×10
Mixed type associating solid, comedo and cribriform patterns.

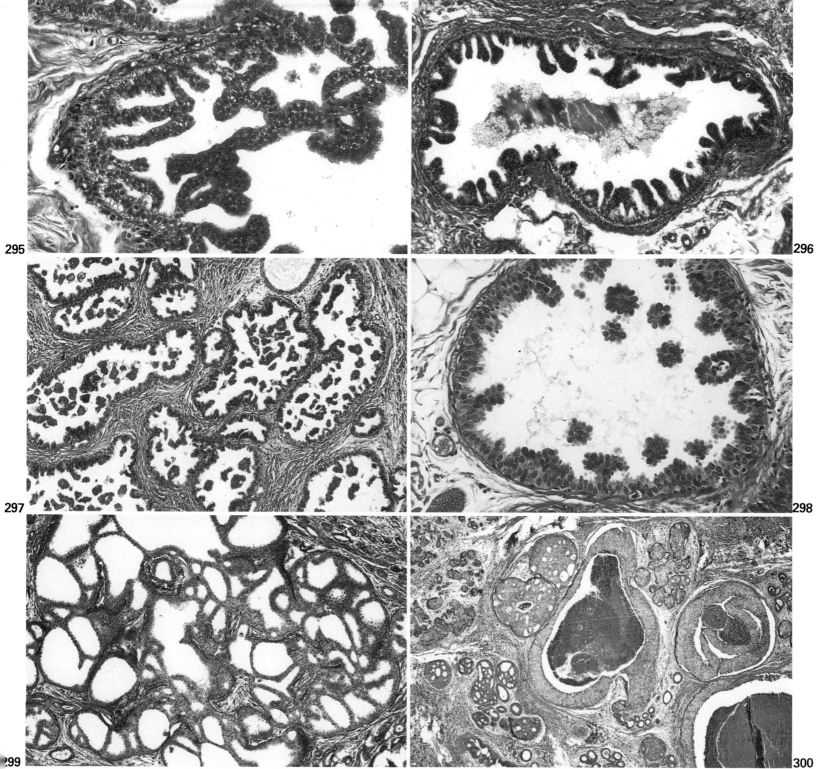

295

296

297

298

299

300

CLINGING TYPE (AZZOPARDI)

Definition

This type of ductal carcinoma in situ must be specially mentioned. Azzopardi isolated it in 1979 and defined it as follows: 'Variant of in situ carcinoma in which ducts keep a visible lumen lined by one, two or just a few layers of epithelial malignant cells. Myoepithelial cells may persist or disappear.'

Site

Predominant in lobules and small ducts.

> • lobular configuration is kept,
> • signs of malignancy are often minimal and more architectural than cytological.

301 HES ×64
302 HES ×160

Clinging carcinoma: epithelium with one cell layer. Note crowding of cells and apical protrusion of some nuclei thrown out in the lumen (hobnail appearance).

303 HES ×64
304 HES ×160

Clinging carcinoma: atypical nuclei, irregular luminal margin.

305 HES ×64
306 HES ×160

Clinging carcinoma: stratified epithelium with apical snouts, loss of nuclei polarity and one mitosis.

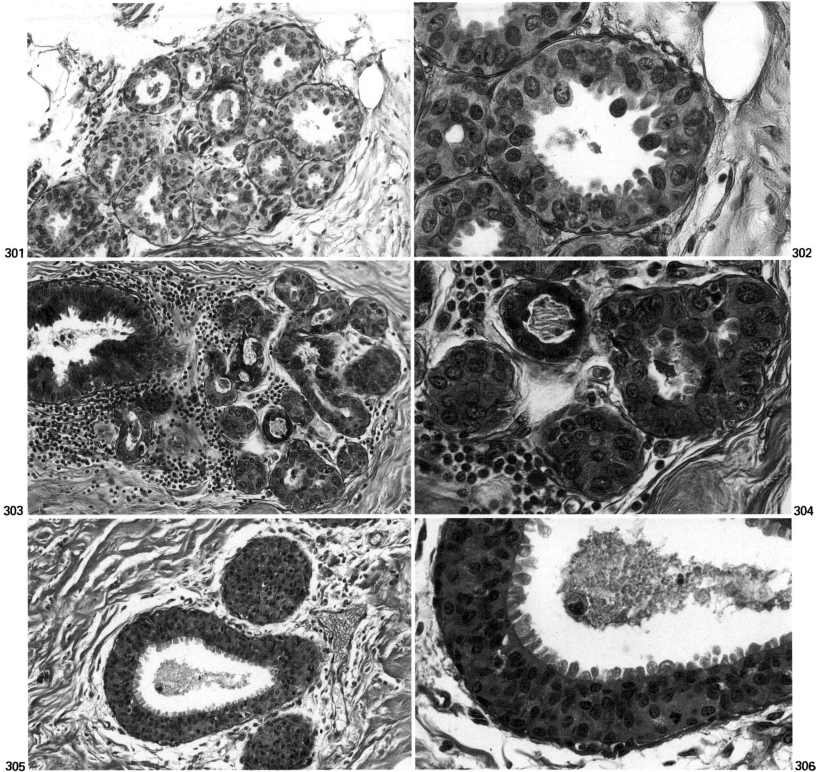

307 HES ×25 ⎫
308 HES ×64 ⎭
Clinging carcinoma: like comedocarcinoma but with sparsity of luminal debris and few cell layers lining the lumen.

309 HES ×25 ⎫
310 HES ×160 ⎭
Clinging carcinoma: a few cribriform or bridging structures; a calcification in a pseudo-papillary epithelial projection.

311 HES ×64 ⎫
312 HES ×160 ⎭
Clinging carcinoma: a few cribriform structures, calcifications within the lumen, epithelium with apical snouts.

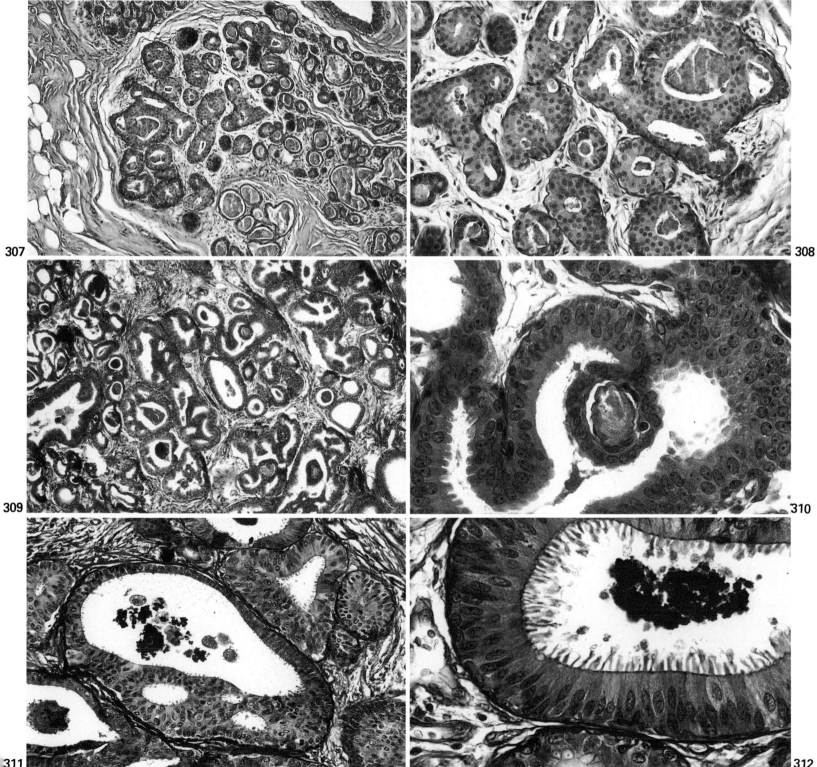

313 HES ×25
314 HES ×64
Clinging carcinoma: 'bridging', i.e. bridge formation spanning the lumen with cells arranged perpendicular to the axis of the bridge.

315 HES ×10
316 HES ×64
Clinging carcinoma: lobular configuration; a few bridge formations only testify to malignancy.

317 HES ×25
318 HES ×160
Clinging carcinoma: in medium-sized ducts, a few bridges and a few short papillary tufts free in the lumen.

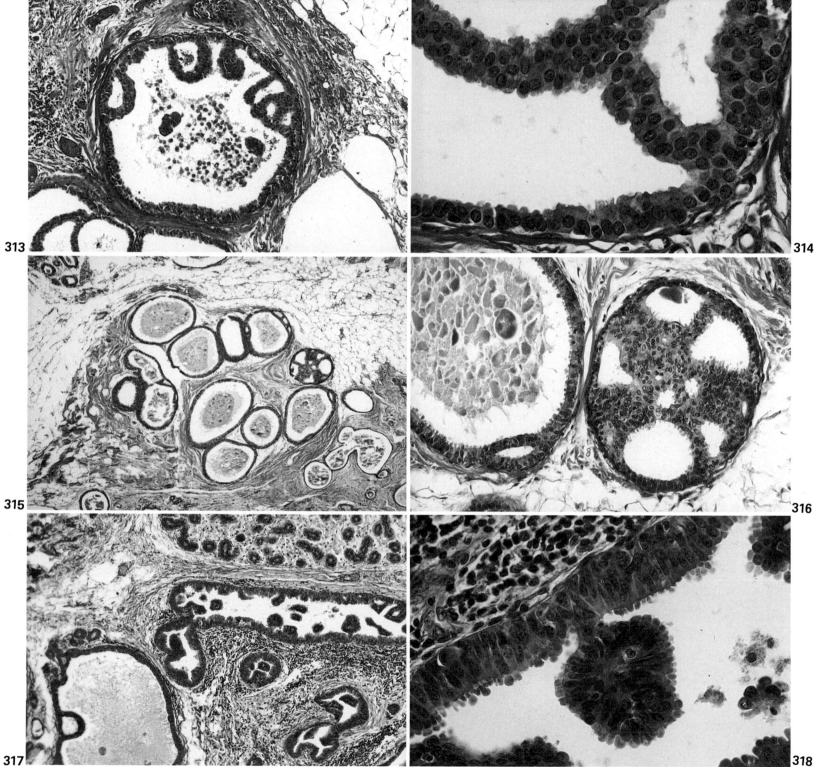

CELL CHARACTERISTICS

All degrees of cell atypia are seen, the most marked in the comedo type. Rounded form and uniformity of nuclei are good criteria of malignancy in small cell ductal carcinoma in situ as opposed to epitheliosis.

319 PAS ×160
Solid type DCIS
320 HES ×160
Comedo type DCIS
Marked cell atypia, frequent mitosis.

321 HES ×160
Large cell cribriform DCIS: round or ovoid nuclei.

322 HES ×160
Large cell cribriform DCIS: cleaved and hyperchromatic nuclei.

323 HES ×160
Small cell cribriform DCIS: round and regular nuclei.

324 HES ×160
Small cell papillary DCIS: ovoid regular nuclei.

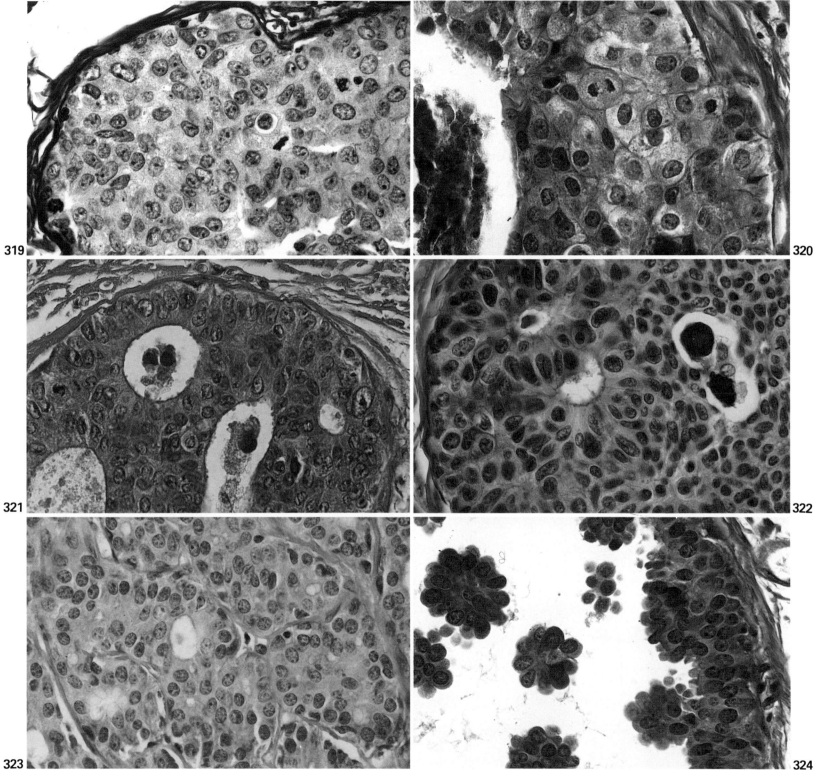

VARIANTS

Non-invasive intracystic carcinoma: corresponds according to WHO to a papillary carcinoma arising in and limited to a mammary cyst.

Apocrine ductal carcinoma in situ: in which cells have apocrine characteristics (acidophile granular cytoplasm with apical granules).

According to Haagensen, these carcinomas probably originate from malignant change of metaplastic apocrine epithelium of cysts or ducts. According to him, apocrine metaplasia in gross cystic disease constitutes a risk factor, a feature not found by other authors.

Mucinous ductal carcinoma in situ: is rarely a pure intraductal form and is generally associated with foci of totally or partially mucinous invasive carcinoma. Ducts have a dilated, mucin-filled lumen with a few bridge structures.

325–326 Non-invasive intracystic carcinoma.

325 Macroscopy
Small rosy tumour implanted within a thick-walled cyst.

326 HES ×25
Thick fibrous wall, cribriform proliferation.

327 HES ×25 ⎫
328 HES ×64 ⎭
Apocrine DCIS

329 Mucicarmin ×25 ⎫
330 Mucicarmin ×160 ⎭
Mucinous DCIS

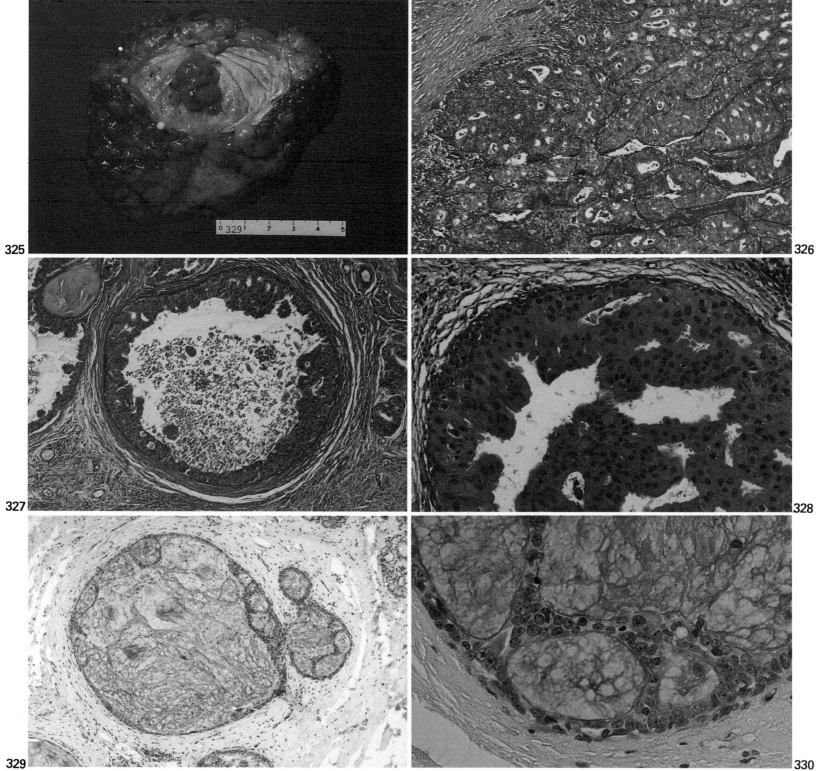

Ductal carcinoma in situ in duct ectasia: arises in pre-existing duct ectasia in atrophic breasts of old women. Diagnosis may be difficult because of the frequent clinging type.

Ductal carcinoma in situ and vessels: Figures 335–336.

331 HES ×10 ⎫
332 HES ×10 ⎪
333 HES ×64 ⎬
334 HES ×160 ⎭
Large duct with changes of pre-existing duct ectasia. Epithelium shows a loss of polarity and anaplasia of cells and a few epithelial projections in the lumen filled with debris.

335 HES ×160 ⎫
336 HES ×160 ⎭
DCIS closely related to periductal capillaries; the basement membrane is sometimes ruptured within a capillary.

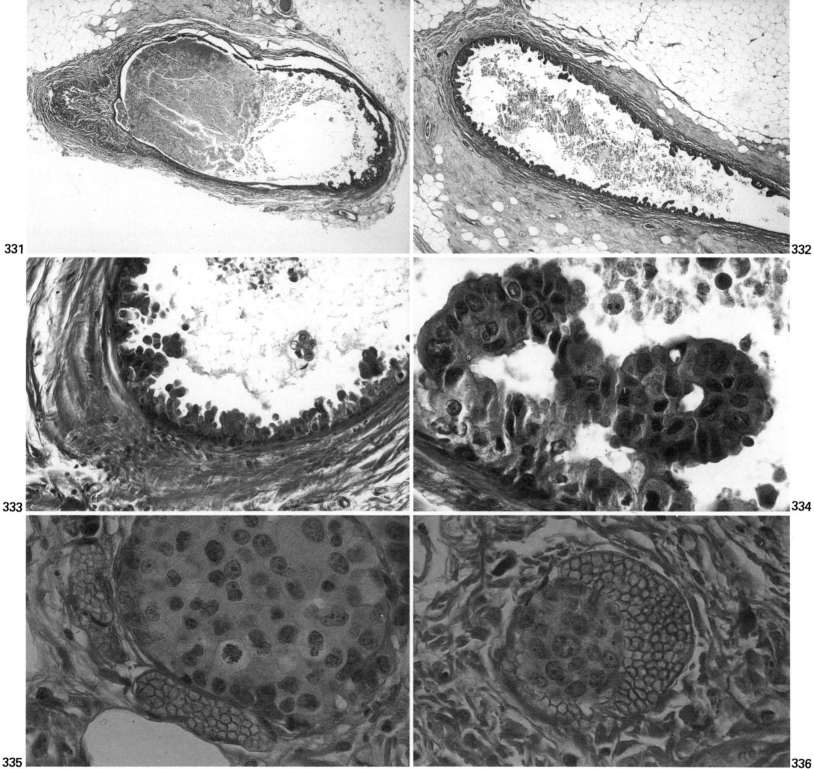

MULTICENTRICITY

Multicentricity of a carcinoma is defined by foci of the same histological type remote from the dominant mass. The meaning of 'remote from' varies between the authors, either >5cm, or in a different quadrant, or without continuity between the dominant mass and second focus.

Fisher (1986) distinguishes multicentricity from multifocality: multifocality corresponds to carcinomatous foci in the vicinity of or within the same quadrant.

The origin of multicentric ductal carcinoma in situ foci is probably both intraductal spread and in situ origin.

Two histological features of the ductal carcinoma in situ extension are frequent:
- lobular cancerization
- pagetoid spread

Lobular cancerization

This term has been used at first to indicate the site of a ductal carcinoma in the lobule by retrograde spread. The term is currently used in cases of ductal carcinoma in situ to indicate localization of the cancer within lobules without presuming its origin. Histological appearances of the 'lobular cancerization' correspond to all growth patterns of ductal carcinoma in situ. However, the 'clinging' type is particularly frequent in this site.

337   PAS ×25
Spread in the lobule of carcinoma with injection of the dilated extralobular terminal duct.

338   HES ×64
Lobular cancerization: the DCIS has a cribriform pattern in the extralobular terminal duct and a 'clinging' pattern in acini.

339   HES ×64
Lobular cancerization: 'clinging' pattern with discrete features of comedo type.

340   HES ×25
Lobular cancerization: solid pattern. Irregular dilatation of filled terminal ductules and inflammatory lobular stroma.

Pagetoid spread: Figures 341–342

341   HES ×64
342   HES ×160
Large atypical cells with prominent nucleoli and pale cytoplasm tend to replace and destroy the overlying epithelium. Diagnosis of DCIS is easy in this case, but sometimes, malignant cells are regular and small and the differential diagnosis with LCIS may be impossible (page 116).

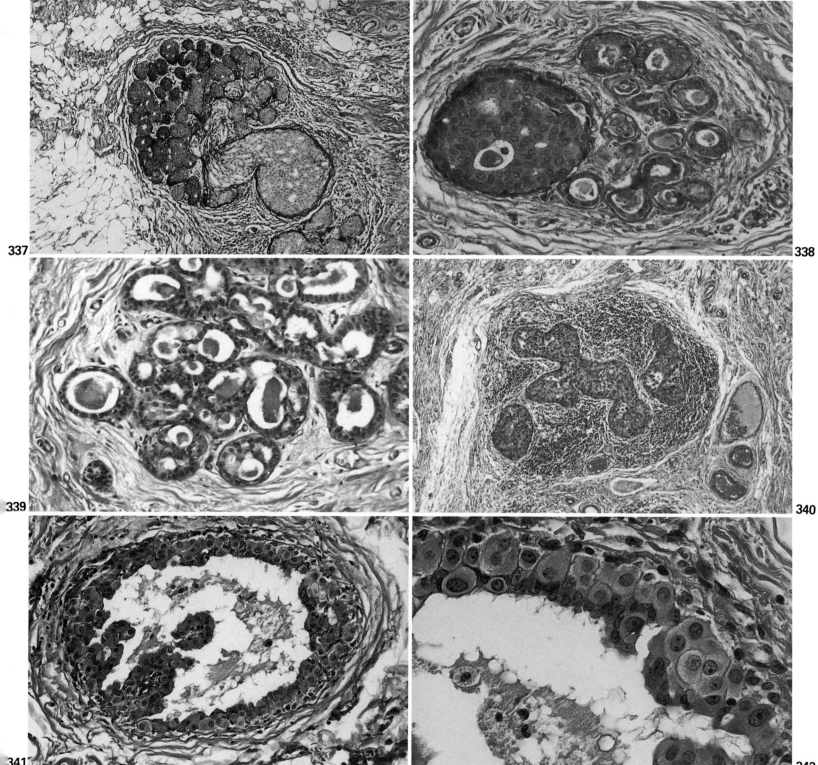

DIFFERENTIAL DIAGNOSIS

With benign lesions

DCIS	Possible lesion	Benign
Papillary DCIS (papillae with fibrous stalk)	Multiple papilloma (possible malignant change)	Papilloma
Papillary DCIS (pseudopapillae without fibrous stalk)		
Solid DCIS	Atypical epitheliosis	Epitheliosis
Cribriform DCIS	Cribriform ADH	
Clinging DCIS		BDA

Some lesions are very difficult to classify between ductal carcinoma in situ and benign epithelial hyperplasia. The problem of the relationship between hyperplasia and carcinoma remains unresolved: it may be a continuous spectrum with intermediate steps, or independent processes without linear histogenetic relationship. In these cases, slides are incapable of showing all the difficulty. Therefore, few examples are shown here.

Atypical ductal hyperplasia (epitheliosis)

343 HES ×25
344 HES ×160

Glandular spaces are irregular and not round but more rigid than in a typical epitheliosis. Cells have nuclei irregular in shape but more voluminous with conspicuous nucleoli than in typical epitheliosis. Note a cluster of foamy histiocytes in the duct centre.

Clinging carcinoma in blunt duct adenosis

345 HES ×10
346 HES ×64

All ducts have a benign appearance except four of them which have a different epithelium with early cribriform pattern, typical of carcinoma (Figure 346). Is it malignant change of BDA or simple coexistence? The question remains unanswered.

347 HES ×64

BDA (late phase); pseudocribriform pattern due to irregular duct contours (to be differentiated from DCIS).

348 HES ×25

In an involutive breast without malignant proliferation, an area of atypical ductal hyperplasia with cribriform pattern (possibly borderline with or corresponding to DCIS).

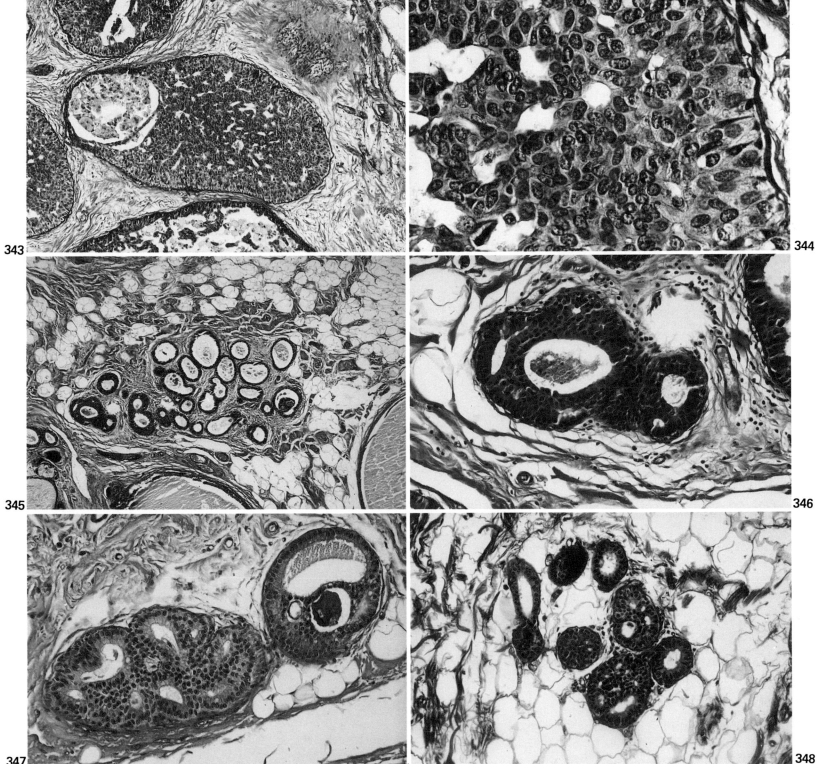

With other malignant lesions

- Lobular carcinoma in situ (page 116)
- Invasive ductal carcinoma with a predominant intraductal component
- Invasive ductal carcinoma
- Adenoid cystic carcinoma (page 188).

With invasive ductal carcinoma with a predominant intraductal component (IDC-pred ID):

Some histological patterns raise the question of the presence or absence of a microinvasive growth:
- lobular cancerization
- 'duct within a duct'
- intraductal fibrosis and necrosis.

349 HES ×25
350 Cytok ×25
351 HES ×64
352 Cytok ×64

Lobular cancerization: acini are filled with DCIS and surrounded by an inflammatory stroma. Two errors are possible:
- either such acini are mistaken for an invasive carcinoma,
- or the diagnosis is 'lobular cancerization in a DCIS' and a microinvasive growth as single cells within the inflammatory stroma may be missed. In this case, epithelial antigen markers help to visualize these cells.

353 HES ×10
354 HES ×10

Appearances of 'duct within a duct' (Cowen) mean infiltrating and not only intraductal growth.

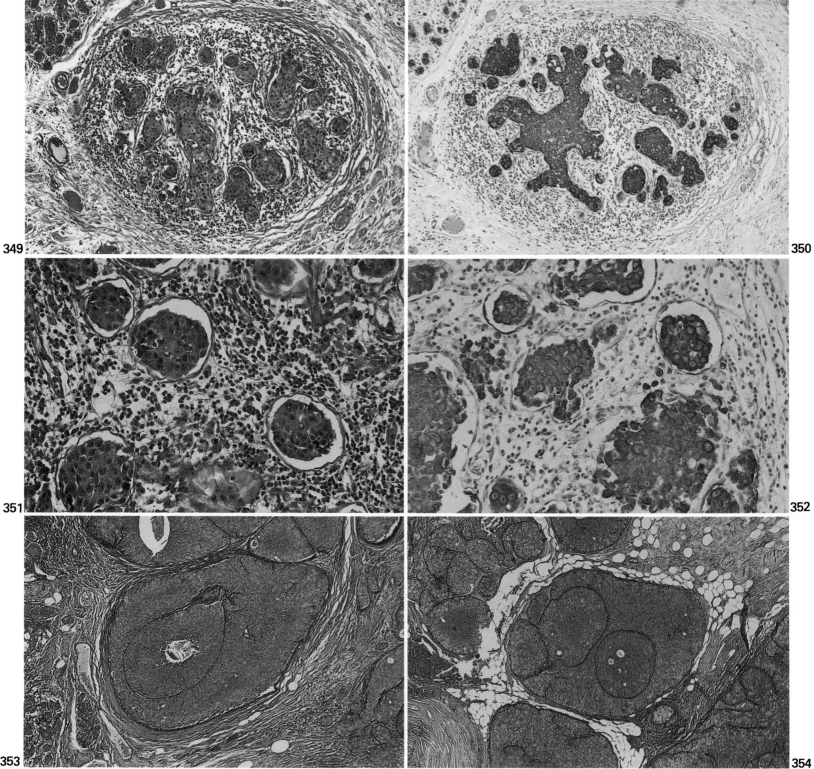

Intraductal proliferation and even the whole duct may disappear because of fibrosis or necrosis. These phenomena are interpreted by Fisher as a regression of carcinoma. Others think that they constitute precursor signs of invasion.

355   HES ×25
The duct wall is circumscribed by an obvious peripheric elastosic tissue. Fibrosis partially obliterates the lumen in which only a few DCIS nests remain.

356   HES ×10
Duct with fibrous invagination in the lumen, irregular contours and altered basement membrane.

357   HES ×25
DCIS is disappearing within fibrosis. A lymphoid infiltrate surrounds the obliterated duct.

358   HES ×25
Total intraductal necrosis with destruction of the duct wall and granulomatous infiltrate around.

359   HES ×10
360   HES ×160
Total necrosis of intraductal proliferation with rupture of the basement membrane, rejection of necrotic debris outside of the ductal lumen and periductal inflammatory reaction.

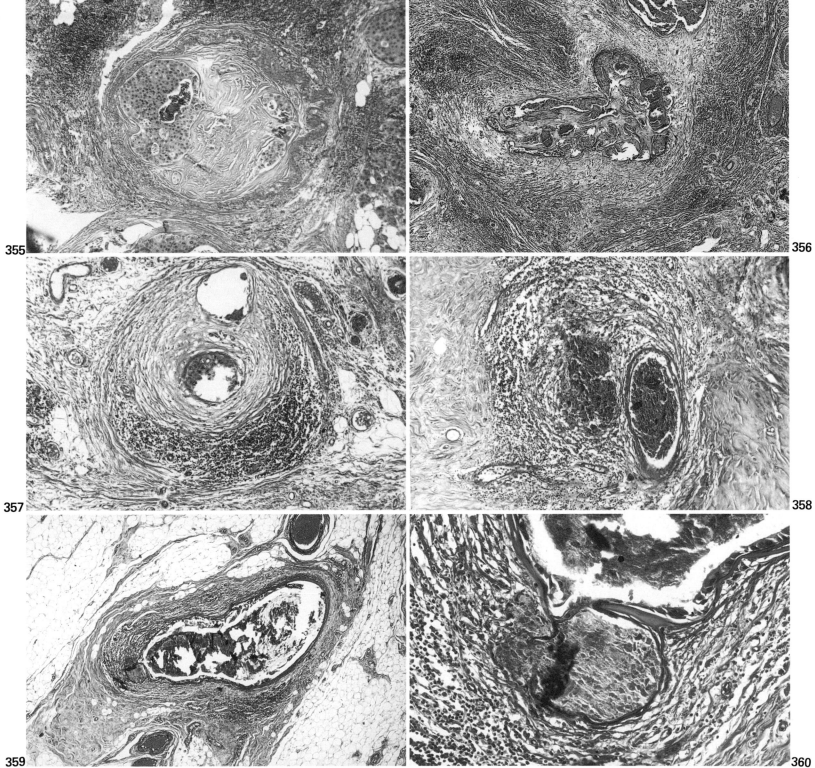

With invasive ductal carcinoma showing intraductal appearances (comedo, papillary or cribriform pattern). Diagnosis of infiltrating growth is certain only if the same intraductal appearances are found in lymph node metastases. A true intraductal component is often associated with this type of carcinoma, the amount of which is impossible to determine. This type of carcinoma might be a ductal carcinoma in situ at the beginning, then become an invasive carcinoma keeping the same architectural pattern.

361 HES ×10
Breast tumour

362 HES ×25
Axillary lymph node:
IDC with central necrosis of trabeculae, resembling a comedo DCIS. The same structures are present in the axillary metastasis.

363 HES ×10
Breast tumour

364 HES ×25
Axillary lymph node:
IDC with tubulopapillary formations like a papillary type DCIS. The same structures are present in the axillary metastasis.

365 HES ×10
Breast tumour

366 HES ×10
Axillary lymph node:
IDC with cart-wheel formations also found in the lymph node.

7.2 INVASIVE CARCINOMA

INVASIVE DUCTAL CARCINOMA (IDC)
NOT OTHERWISE SPECIFIED (NOS)

Definition

'Invasive carcinoma not falling into any of the other categories with possible foci of intraductal carcinoma.'

Nosology

This tumour has been referred to as infiltrating duct carcinoma with productive fibrosis. Linell (1980) has divided the invasive ductal carcinoma group into the two subgroups of tubuloductal carcinoma and ductal carcinoma of comedo type. He has individualized these two categories to provide a better prognostic prediction because 'a classification where 70–85% of the tumours comprise one major group has little value for prognostic prediction'.

Tubuloductal carcinoma

- origin in the centre of a radial scar and progression from tubular to lesser differentiated forms
- no intraductal growth
- no lobular cancerization
- absence of Paget's disease
- remnants of scar with elastosis
- most often small cells
- a prognosis much better than the following type.

Ductal carcinoma of comedo type

- origin in the TDLU
- intraductal growth (all patterns)
- lobular cancerization
- possibility of Paget's disease
- no remnants of scar
- large cells
- a prognosis worse than the type.

But these histogenetic theories are controversial and denied by many authors.

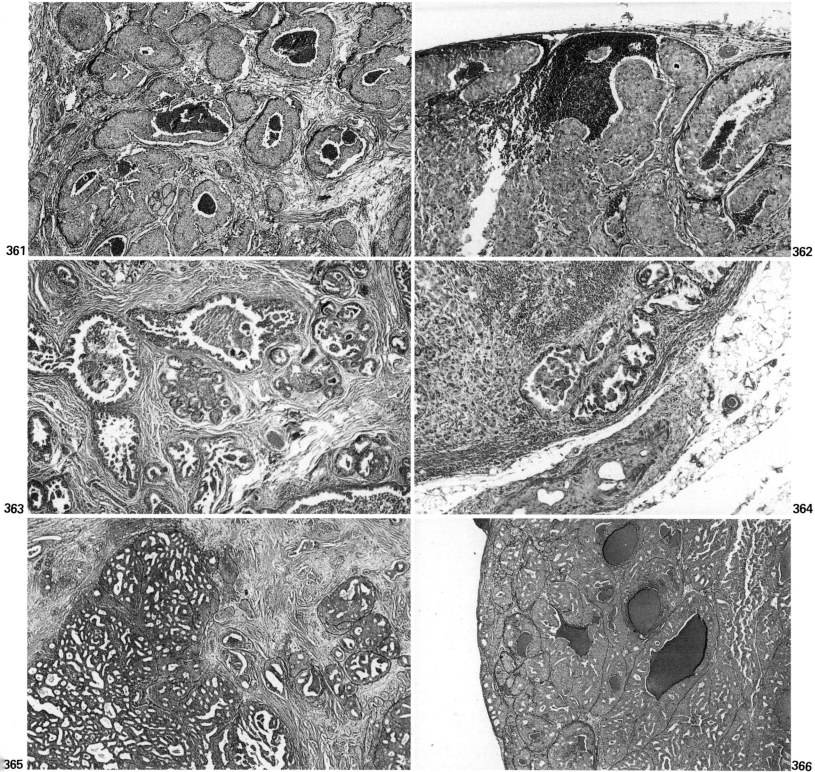

Clinical features

- frequent form: 70%,
- detection: palpable tumour, rarely only mammographic signs,
- age: two peaks, pre- and postmenopausal,
- site: predominance in the upper outer quadrant,
- bilaterality: 5 to 8%,
- multicentricity: 15 to 20%,
- metastatic axillary lymph nodes: 40 to 50%.

Histological features

- contours: stellate or irregular, circumscribed or lobulated,
- growth pattern: well differentiated, moderately differentiated, undifferentiated: according to the relative amounts of tubules and trabeculae,
- intraductal component (page 000), present in 75% cases.

Prognostic factors

- tumour size,
- number of metastatic axillary lymph nodes,
- histologic grade,
- hormonal receptor content within the tumour.

CONTOURS

- well-defined or circumscribed, rounded or lobulated, 'pushing' the surrounding tissue, sometimes forming a fibrous pseudocapsule;

- irregular or stellate with radial projections, 'infiltrating' the surrounding tissue;

- both pushing and infiltrating type of growth according to areas.

Divergent results have been noted with regard to the relationship between circumscription and prognosis. These divergences are probably due either to medullary forms included in the group studied or to different methods of evaluation of tumour borders.

Comparative examination of tumour on mammogram, surgical specimen, and mount section.

Stellate form
case 1: **367–369**
case 2: **370–372**
In both two cases, we find a stellate tumour: spicules radiating in the surrounding tissue, very hard consistency.

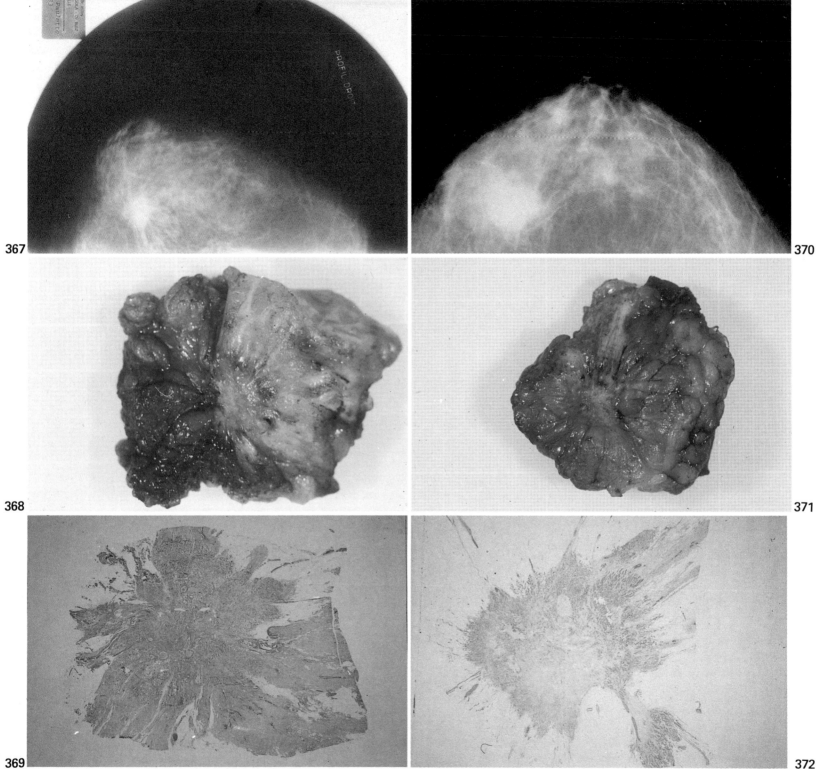

367

370

368

371

369

372

Circumscribed form: case 3

373 Mammography
round tumour with sharply outlined contours, without signs of malignancy.

374 Macroscopy
the cut surface is soft with suspicious central necrosis.

375 HES ×25
fibrous pseudocapsule surrounding the proliferation.

Circumscribed form with focal infiltration: case 4

376 Mammography
rounded tumour, suspicious because of an irregular posterior border.

377 Macroscopy
well-circumscribed nodule, with soft and bright cut surface.

378 HES ×5
carcinoma with inflammatory stroma and focal peripheral infiltration.

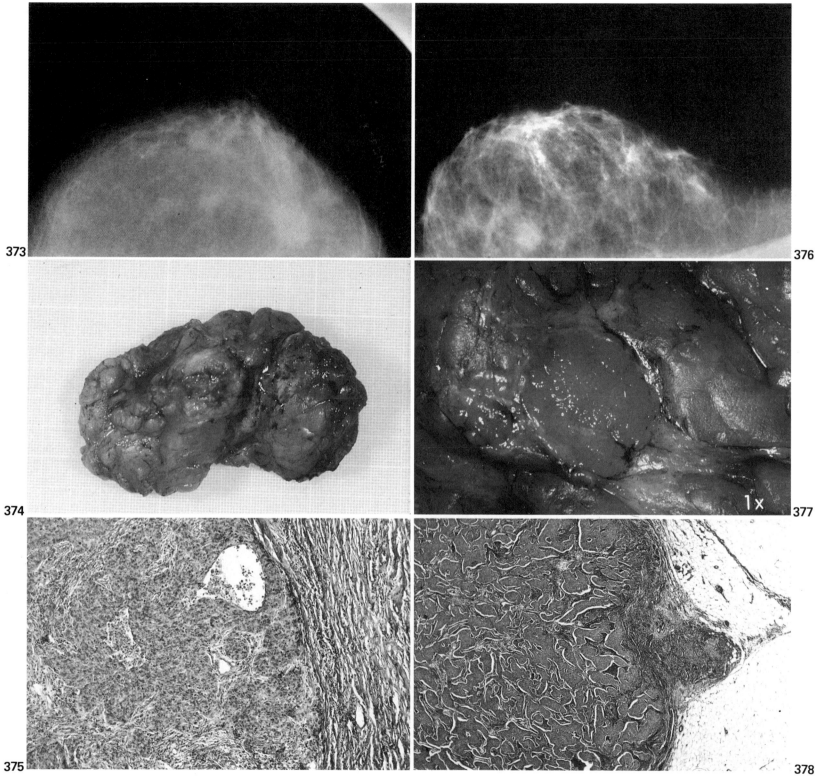

Circumscribed form with focal infiltration: case 5

379 Mammography
round tumour with anterior well-defined and posterior irregular contours.

380 Macroscopy
round, well-circumscribed tumour, with soft and hemorrhagic cut surface.

381 HES ×25
well-delimited part, with pseudocapsule punctuated by abundant hemosiderin deposits.

382 HES ×25
area of infiltration of adipose tissue.

Circumscribed form: cases 6 and 7

383 HES ×1 ⎫
384 HES ×1 ⎭
mount sections of two tumours with well-circumscribed, lobulated contours.

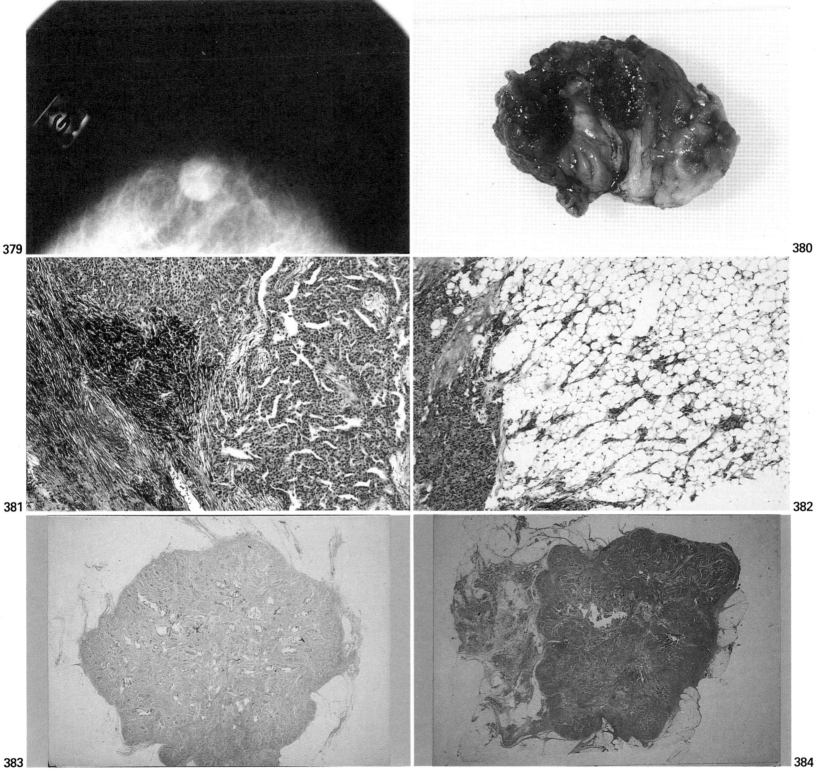

379

380

381

382

383

384

HISTOLOGICAL GRADING

Histological grading of breast carcinomas has proved to be useful in evaluating prognosis. The most employed system is that of Bloom and Richardson, see diagram below, according to criteria given by the authors.

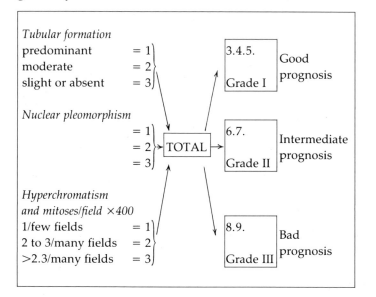

Criticisms

- low reproducibility: particularly because of very personal adaptation of ill-defined criteria.
- the same weight is arbitrarily given to each of the three parameters in the gradation.

However, a relationship between histologic grade and prognosis is always found because histologic factors related to the tumour growth occur (differentiation, mitoses).

Other systems have been used such as Black's (1957) based on nuclear grade (grade 1 the worst).

Their reproducibility is not better.

Differentiation

Corresponds to the tubular formation, clearer in the centre of the tumour than in the periphery.

385 HES ×25: = *1*
Tubules are predominant.

386 HES ×25: = *2*
Mixture of tubules and trabeculae.

387 HES ×25: = *2*
Cribriform pattern.

388 HES ×25: = *3*
Trabecular or solid areas without tubules.

389 HES ×160
Adipose vacuoles inside a carcinomatous nest; to be distinguished from a glandular structure.

390 HES ×160
Artefactual slits or holes due to necrosis without polarity of cells around the lumen; to be distinguished from true glands.

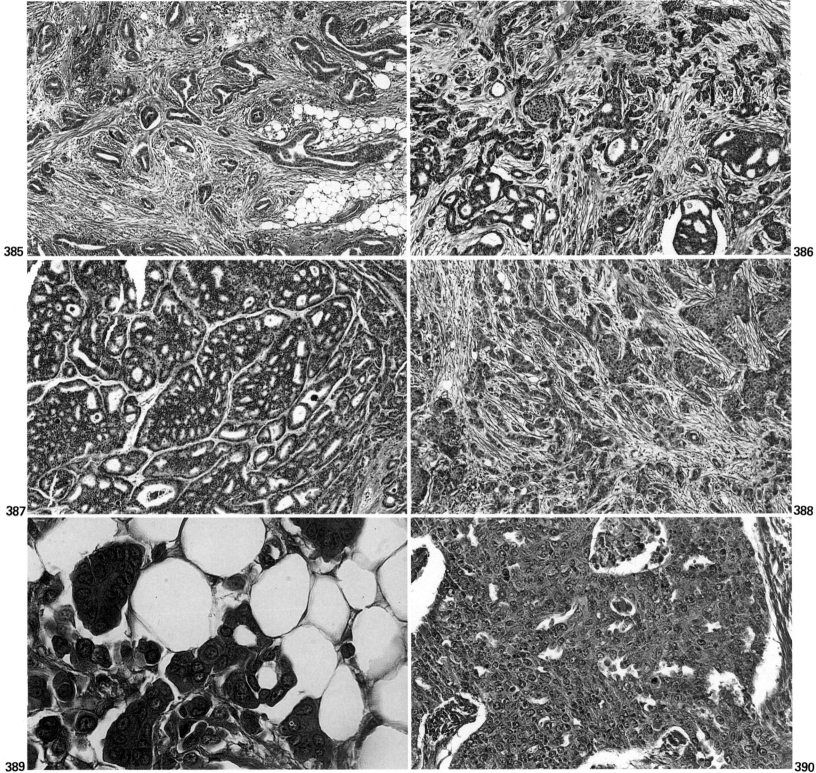

385

386

387

388

389

390

Nuclear pleomorphism

This criterion is very subjective and variable from one observer to another.

> Note: it is more important to take into account the differences in size and shape of the nuclei with regard to each other, rather than their absolute size, even if the nuclei are quite large.

391 HES ×160 ⎫
392 HES ×160 ⎭ = *1: discrete pleomorphism*
When all the cells are of comparable size, shape and chromatism and are almost identical to normal epithelial cells.

393 HES ×160 = *2: moderate pleomorphism*

394 HES ×160 = *2: apocrine cells.* Large cells with prominent nucleoli but monotonous size and conservation of N/C ratio.

395 HES ×160 ⎫
396 HES ×160 ⎭ = *3: marked pleomorphism*
Nuclei very irregular in size and shape with multilobulated and giant forms.

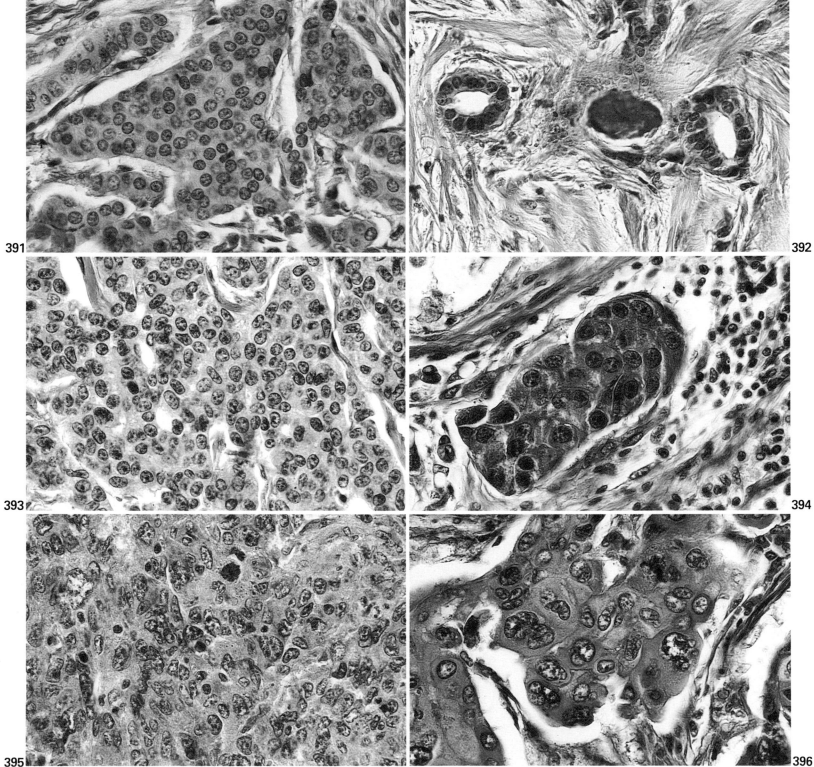

391

392

393

394

395

396

Histologic grade

The authors have studied a series of 1409 cases distributed as follows: 26% grade I, 45% grade II, 29% grade III.

397 HES ×64
Grade I (1 + 2 + 1)

398 HES ×64
Grade I (3 + 1 + 1)

399 HES ×64
400 HES ×160
Grade II (3 + 2 + 1)

401 HES ×64
402 HES ×160
Grade III (3 + 3 + 3)

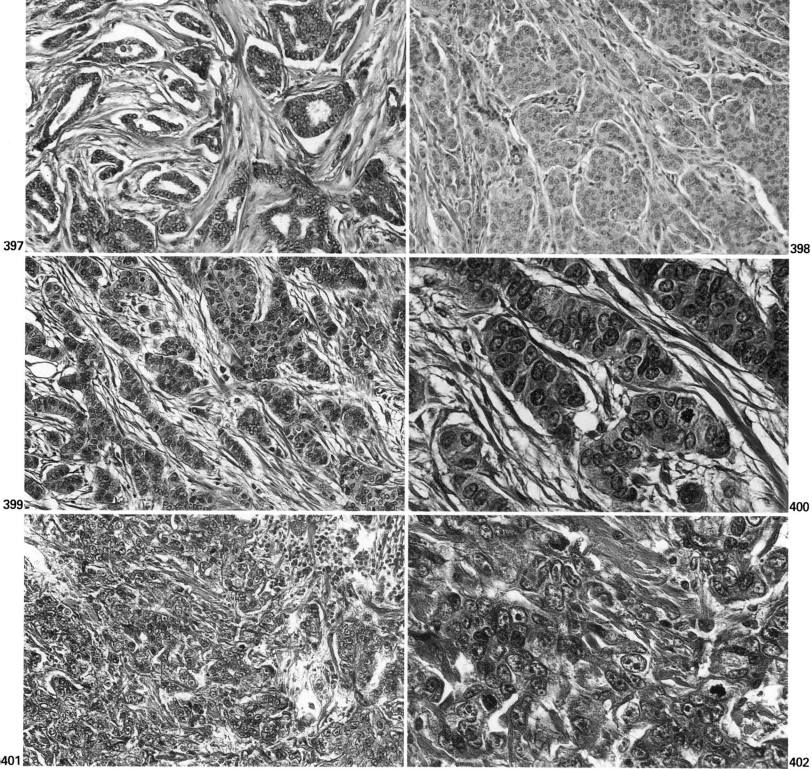

STROMA

Fibrosis and elastosis

Fibrosis is present in almost all breast carcinomas as a stroma-reaction. Fisher divides carcinomas with fibrosis or 'scar cancers' into five groups on the basis of the fibrosis distribution.

Elastosis may be periductal, perivascular or stromal. The first two types affect pre-existing structures. Elastin has been related to estrogen receptor content, tumour differentiation, parity, radiotherapy and chemotherapy. However, it is of no demonstrable prognostic significance. It is probably synthesized by mesenchymal cells (fibroblasts, myofibroblasts and smooth muscle cells). Epithelial cells might stimulate this synthesis but their real role is unknown.

403 HES ×25
Hyaline interstitial sclerosis, punctuated with calcifications.

404 HES ×64
Cellular fibrosis with many fibroblasts.

405 HES ×25
406 HES ×64
Stromal elastosis associated with sclerosis.

407 HES ×64
Periductal elastosis (more marked in the cancerous than in the normal breast). The duct within the tumour has a hyperplastic but not neoplastic epithelium.

408 HES ×25
Marked perivascular elastosis in an invasive ductal carcinoma.

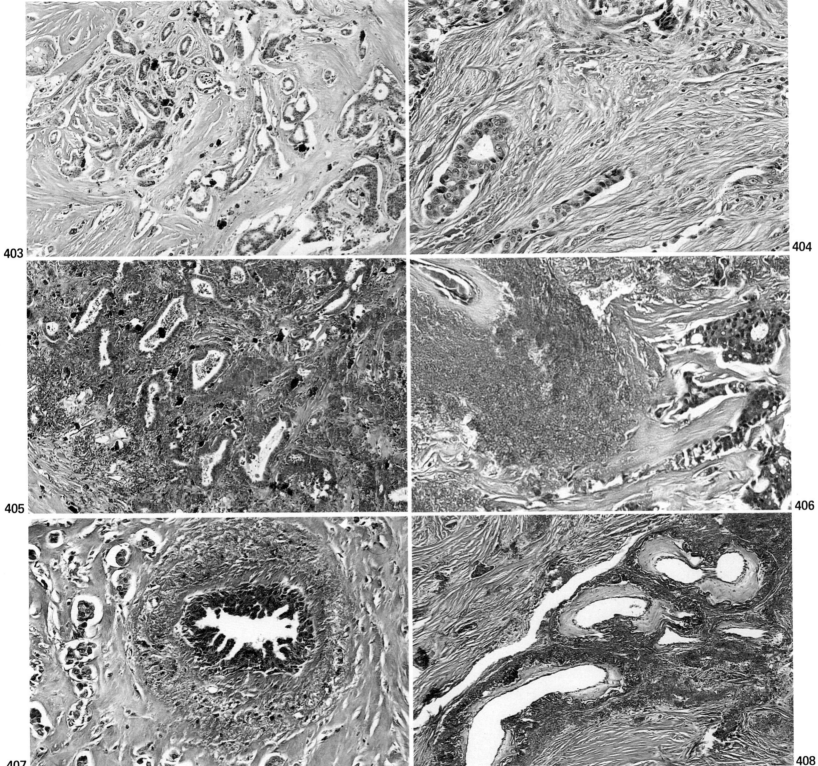

403

404

405

406

407

408

Inflammation

A diffuse lymphoid infiltrate is often associated with a high-grade carcinoma and constitutes in invasive ductal carcinoma a bad prognostic factor. A few carcinomas are associated with histiocytic, sarcoid or giant cell reactions (Chapter 7, page 198).

409 HES ×25 ⎫
410 HES ×25 ⎭ dense lymphoid infiltrate

Dense peripheral lymphoid infiltrate: primary tumour or lymph node metastasis? The differential diagnosis may be very difficult if the tumour is situated in the axillary tail.

Here, a remaining duct proves the primary mammary origin.

411 HES ×25
Diffuse dense lymphoid infiltrate within the tumour.

412 HES ×64
Marked sarcoid reaction in the carcinoma. Similar reactions may be found in axillary lymph nodes. A true sarcoidosis must be eliminated, but breast involvement is very unusual in sarcoidosis and is generally associated with a more diffuse involvement whose diagnosis is known.

413 PAS ×160
PAS-positive histiocytes within the glandular lumina.

414 HES ×64
Multinucleated giant cells are in close contact with the carcinoma.

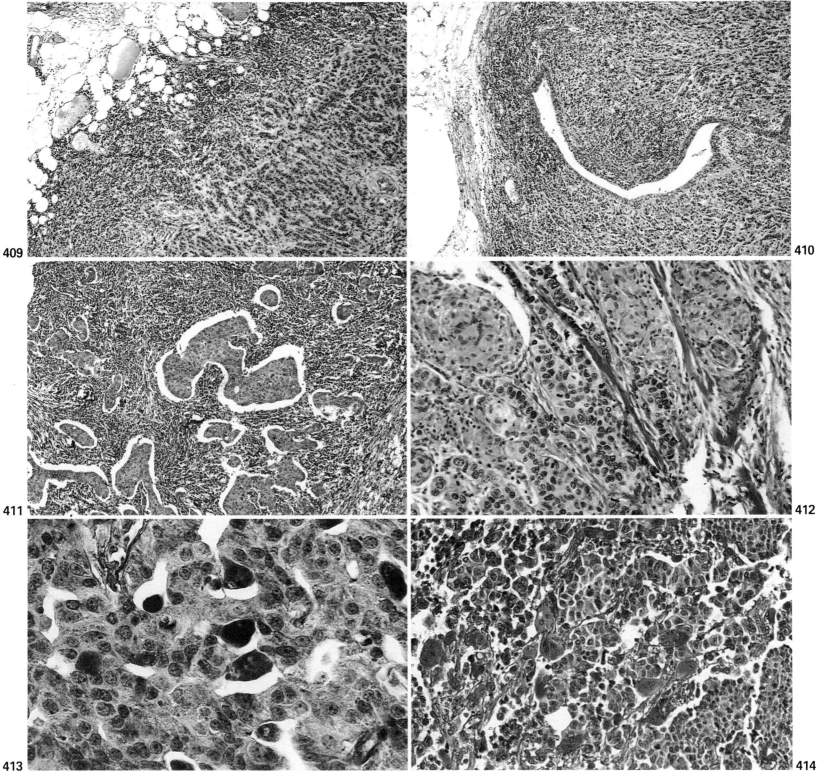

409

410

411

412

413

414

HISTOCHEMISTRY

Glycogen is present in 60% of invasive ductal carcinoma and not related to the degree of differentiation or prognosis.

The mucin is present in most of breast carcinomas, staining with mucicarmine, PAS and alcian blue. The histological type depends on the site and amount of mucin (see diagram below).

Intracytoplasmic mucin vacuoles (target-like) are present in 60% of breast carcinomas (in almost all lobular carcinomas, in 45% of ductal carcinomas) not related to differentiation. They are not specific of the mammary origin of a carcinoma but are more frequently associated with this than any other origin.

Argyrophil cells (detected by the Grimelius staining) are present in 3 to 10% of carcinomas of all histologic types (more frequently in mucinous carcinomas). Argyrophilia alone cannot support the diagnosis of a true carcinoid tumour, rare in the breast and usually associated with production of polypeptide hormones by neoplastic cells.

Currently, immunohistochemical techniques detect antigens or particular constituents on normal or malignant cells and may help to make a diagnosis.
- epithelial antigens, cytoplasmic (cytokeratins) or membranous (EMA).
- vimentin: present in mesenchymal cells.
- leucocyte common antigen: marker of lymphoid cells.
- S100 protein present in myoepithelial and melanocytic cells and nerve fibres.
- GCDFP-15 protein, a marker of the apocrine differentiation.

The list is not exhaustive. There is not yet a specific marker of the lobular or ductal nature of a carcinoma.

415 PAS ×64
Numerous cytoplasmic granules in tumour cells, corresponding to glycogen.

416 PAS ×160
Glycogen condensed along the cytoplasmic membrane.

417 HES ×160
Target-like vacuoles visible by routine staining.

418 D-PAS ×160
Very numerous intracytoplasmic vacuoles in an invasive ductal carcinoma.

419 Grimelius ×160
Small black intracytoplasmic granules.

420 Cytok ×64
Strong positivity of carcinomatous trabeculae.

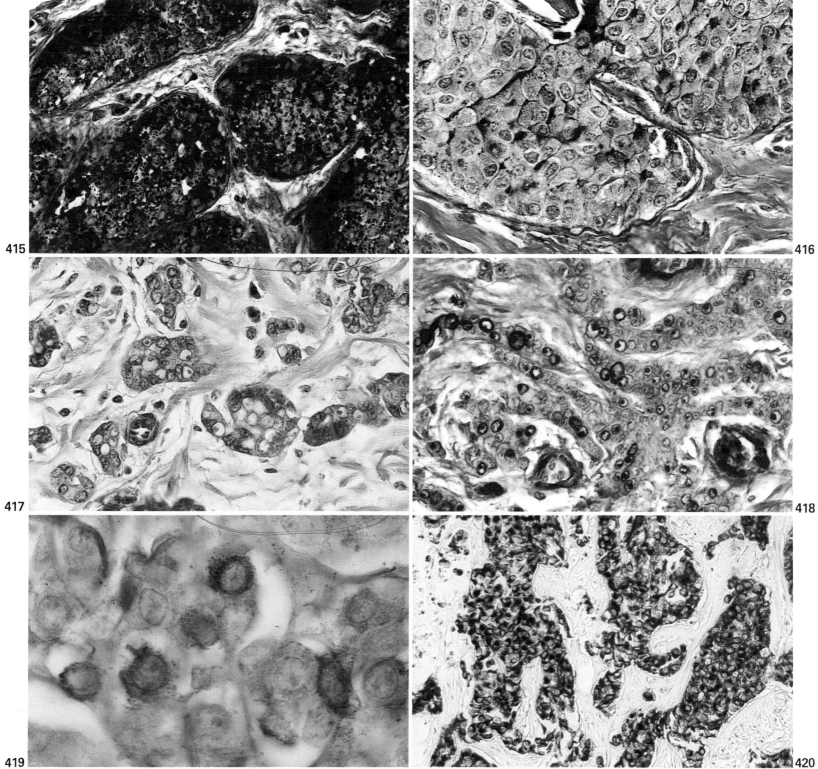

LOCAL TUMOUR EXTENSION

Normal epithelial structures of breast may be penetrated by carcinoma before total destruction. Thus there are possible patterns of pagetoid spread, intraductal or lobular growth.

Carcinoma may also invade blood or lymphatic vessels, perineural spaces and sometimes skeletal myofibres.

421 HES ×64
Pagetoid spread in the ductal epithelium.

422 HES ×64
Early duct involvement.

423 HES ×25
Duct is almost totally obliterated with only a part of its wall remaining.

424 HES ×64
Total obliteration of several ducts but the myo-epithelial cell layer remains.

425 HES ×25
Intraductal propagation and partial lobular involvement.

426 HES ×25
Focal infiltration within lobular stroma with persistence of small acini.

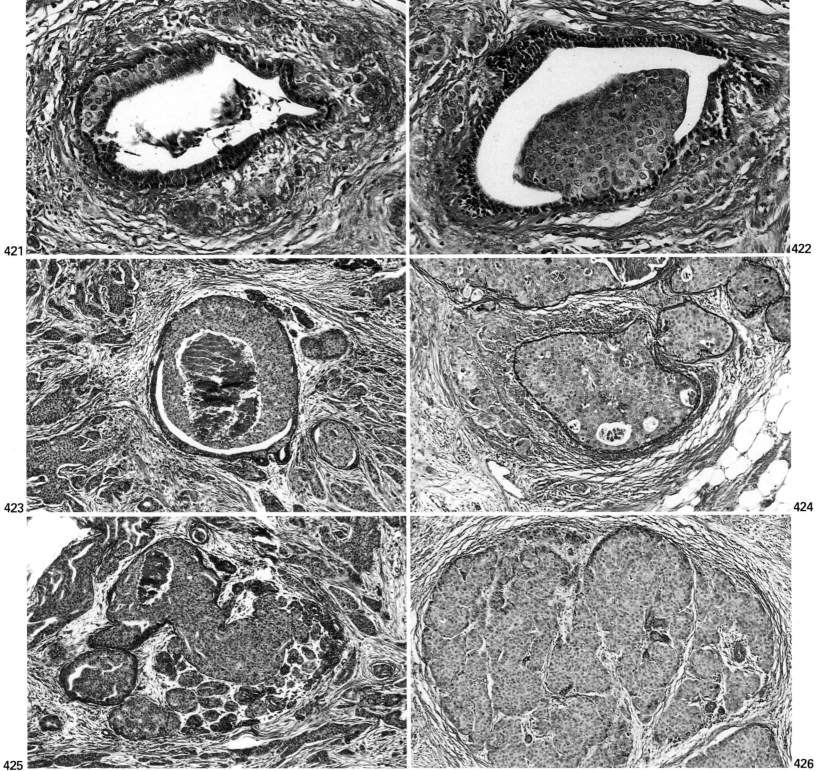

VASCULAR, NERVOUS AND MUSCULAR INVASION

Lymphatic invasion is very difficult to identify within the tumour where it may be simulated by retraction of carcinomatous trabeculae. Lymphatic invasion is more obvious at the periphery, in normal tissue or near a group of vessels.

Lymphatic invasion as a prognostic factor is questionable because of difficulties in identification and low interobserver reproducibility.

427 HES ×25
Lymphatic invasion in mammary tissue around the tumour.

428 HES ×64
Pseudopapillary pattern of lymphatic invasion. This frequent feature must be distinguished from papillary intraductal growth.

429 HES ×25
Venous invasion with infiltration and partial destruction of its wall.

430 HES ×64
Perineural space invasion by an invasive ductal carcinoma.

431 HES ×25
432 HES ×160
Skeletal myofibre invasion: the fibre centre is occupied by carcinoma with a thin peripheral border of sarcolemna.

INVASIVE DUCTAL CARCINOMA WITH A PREDOMINANT INTRADUCTAL COMPONENT

Seventy-five per cent of invasive ductal carcinoma have an intraductal component. It may mean that:
- the invasive process is secondary to the neoplastic progression of the ductal carcinoma in situ. Whether all ductal carcinomas have an in situ stage is questionable. Supporters of this theory think that when ductal carcinoma in situ develops in TDLU, small terminal ducts are rapidly obliterated and may be obscured by progression into invasive cancer. Ductal carcinoma in situ of large ducts should remain purely intraductal for a long time, or .
- the intraductal component is only a stage of carcinomatous spread in ducts at the periphery of or within the tumour. Such patterns have been observed (see page 166).

> **Nevertheless, the more marked the intraductal component, the more probable is the origin from a ductal carcinoma, first in situ, later invasive.**

In bilateral carcinomas, an intraductal component is the essential feature required for the tumour to be considered as a primary neoplasm, rather than a metastasis of the first cancer.

Quantification: the percentage of the intraductal component is always difficult to estimate because it depends on many factors: the subjective character of appreciation, the number of examined tumour sections, the intraductal appearances of a few invasive ductal carcinoma. Two categories are proposed on the basis of relative amounts of the noninvasive and invasive components:
- *Microinvasive intraductal carcinoma*
  the invasive component is very small, defined either by the percentage of tumour surface (<5 or 10%) or by the measure of the greatest diameter (<1mm).

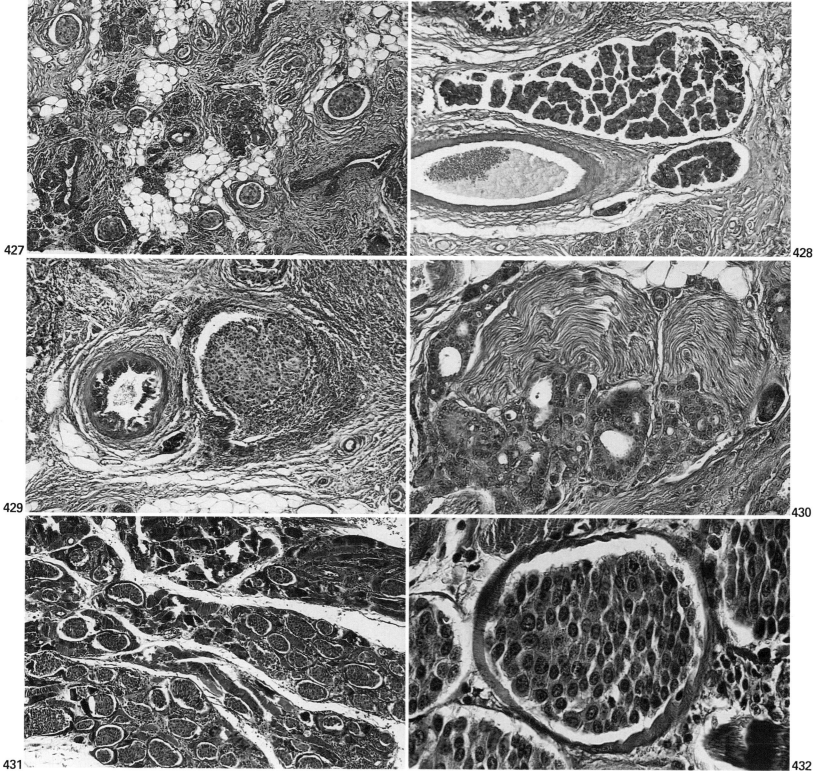

427

428

429

430

431

432

- *Invasive ductal carcinoma with a predominant intraductal component* (invasive ductal carcinoma – pred. IC):

defined by WHO as 'a carcinoma in which the amount of the intraductal carcinoma is at least four times greater than that of the invasive component' (i.e. ⩾80%). This category corresponds to infiltrating comedocarcinoma according to McDivitt (1968) (in which the amount of the intraductal component is not indicated), to ductal carcinoma of comedo type according to Linell (1980), to both subgroups, i.e. infiltrating comedocarcinoma and cribriform carcinoma according to Azzopardi (1979).

Differential diagnosis

microinvasive ductal carcinoma is to be differentiated

- from lobular cancerization (see page 142)
- from appearances of regression (see page 144)
- invasive ductal carcinoma with a predominant intraductal component is to be differentiated from invasive ductal carcinoma with intraductal appearances (see page 146).

Comparative examination of two tumours with a marked intraductal component on mammogram, surgical specimen and histologic slide.

Case 1

433 Mammography
Tumour with irregular contours, spicules and many calcifications.

434 Macroscopy
Ill-defined, firm tumour with many comedones.

435 HES ×10
Intraductal component = 50%.

Case 2 Microinvasive carcinoma

436 Mammography
Microcalcifications scattered from nipple to outer mammary region, ending in cystic pictures.

437 Macroscopy
Within cystic formations, whitish granular vegetations or hemorrhagic fluid.

438 HES ×10
Cyst formation with thick fibrous wall and intraluminal proliferation. The microinvasive process is not visible here.

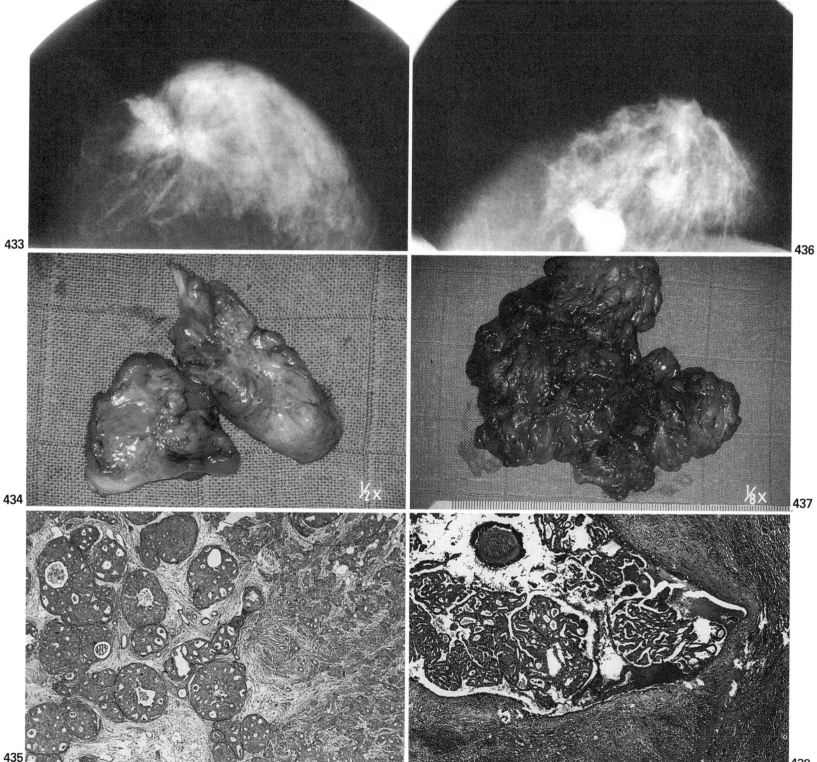

433

436

434

½x

437

⅛x

435

438

The histological appearances of the intraductal component are similar to the growth patterns of ductal carcinoma in situ.

439   HES ×25
Intraductal component of comedo type.

440   HES ×25
Cribriform intraductal component.

441   HES ×10
442   HES ×25
Mixed intraductal component.

443   HES ×25
Mucinous intraductal component with a micro-invasive nest.

444   HES ×25
Intraductal component of comedo type: disrupted duct wall and small invasive nests around an inflammatory granuloma.

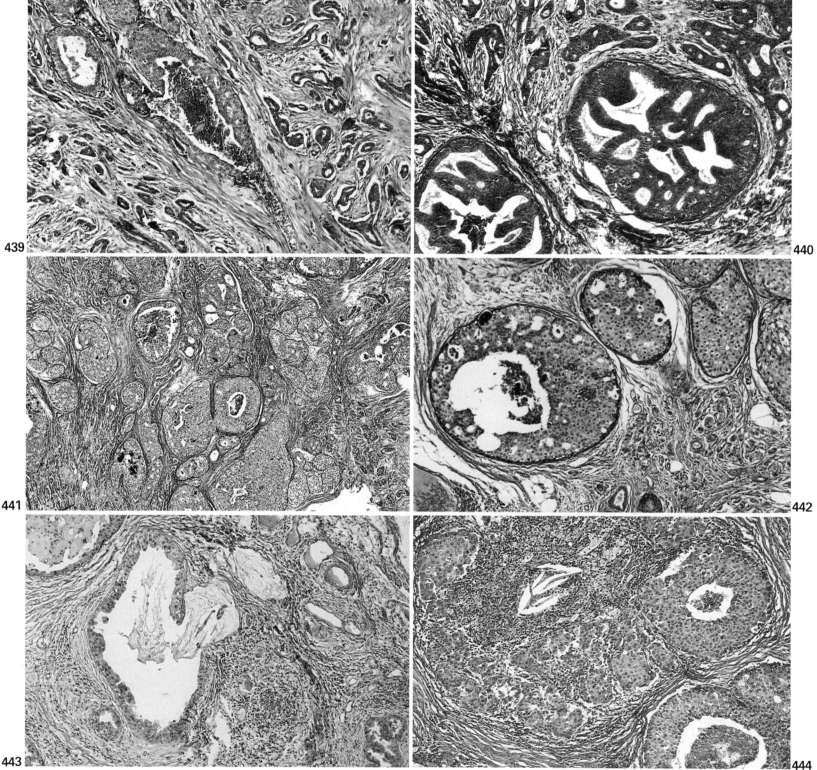

INVASIVE LOBULAR CARCINOMA (ILC)

Definition

'An invasive carcinoma composed of uniform cells resembling those of lobular carcinoma in situ and usually having a low mitotic rate.'

Clinical features

- Frequency: 5 to 15% of cancers.
- Detection: ill-defined tumour mass, sometimes no radiological signs.
- Bilaterality and multicentricity similar to lobular carcinoma in situ.

Histological features

- Associated with lobular carcinoma in situ in 70% of cases
- Typical form: tumour cells are single, in Indian file or arranged concentrically around ducts in a target-like pattern. They are regular with intracytoplasmic mucinous inclusions.
- Variants: trabecular, solid, tubulolobular (Fisher), alveolar, 'signet-ring cell', histiocytoid types.

Differential diagnosis

- Invasive ductal carcinoma. This may be very difficult in variants of invasive ductal carcinoma. No immunohistochemical marker allows up to now to differentiate the ductal or lobular origin of a carcinoma.
- Non-Hodgkin malignant lymphoma: within the tumour or lymph node metastases (Chapter 9).

ILC – Typical form

445 HES ×64
Targetoid pattern of infiltration around ducts.

446 HES ×64 ⎫
447 HES ×160 ⎭
Single or in 'Indian file' cells.

ILC – Pseudolymphomatous appearance

448 HES ×64 ⎫
449 PAS-D ×400 ⎬
450 Cytok ×160 ⎭
Adipose tissue infiltrated by single cells without fibrous stroma-reaction. The diagnosis of lymphoma has to be rejected because of intracytoplasmic mucinous vacuoles, epithelial antigen positivity and leucocyte common antigen negativity.

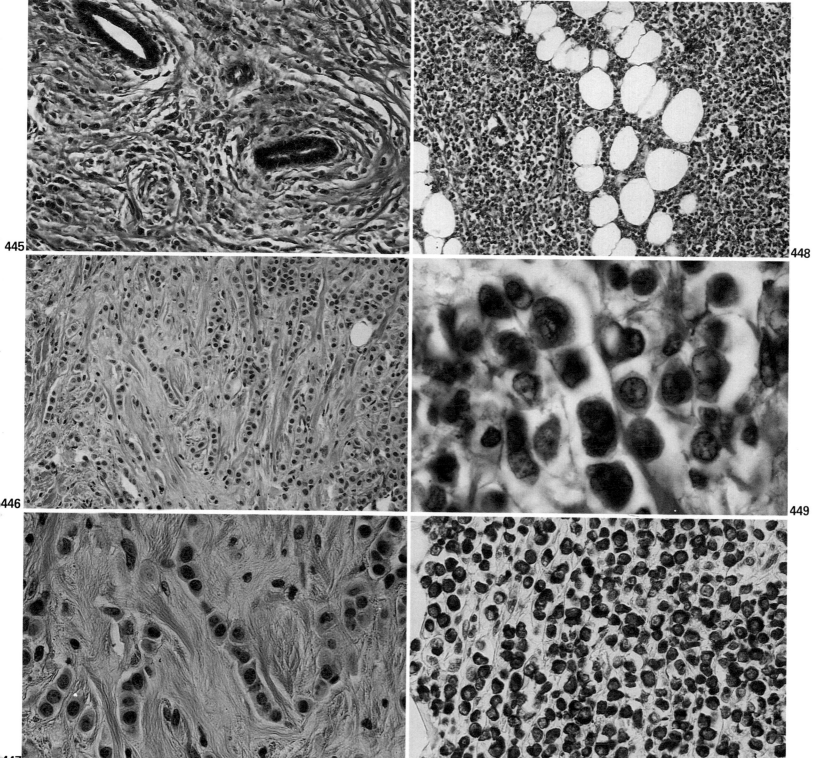

445

448

446

449

447

450

451 AB-PAS ×400
Intracytoplasmic mucinous vacuole:
- alcianophilic blue halo due to predominance of acid mucosaccharides (sialomucine)
- central eosinophilic core of neutral mucosaccharides stained with PAS.

452 HES ×160
ILC cells are not as regular and typical as is usually stated. Note frequent cleaved nuclei. Atypical nuclei can lead to misgivings about lobular origin of carcinoma.

ILC – Variants

453 HES ×64
Trabecular type.
Most of the trabeculae are two or three cells thick.

454 HES ×64
Solid type.
Sheet-like pattern or irregularly shaped nests of closely aggregated cells.

455 HES ×25
456 HES ×160
Tubulolobular type of Fisher.
Presence in an otherwise typical ILC of tubules with closed or almost closed lumina.

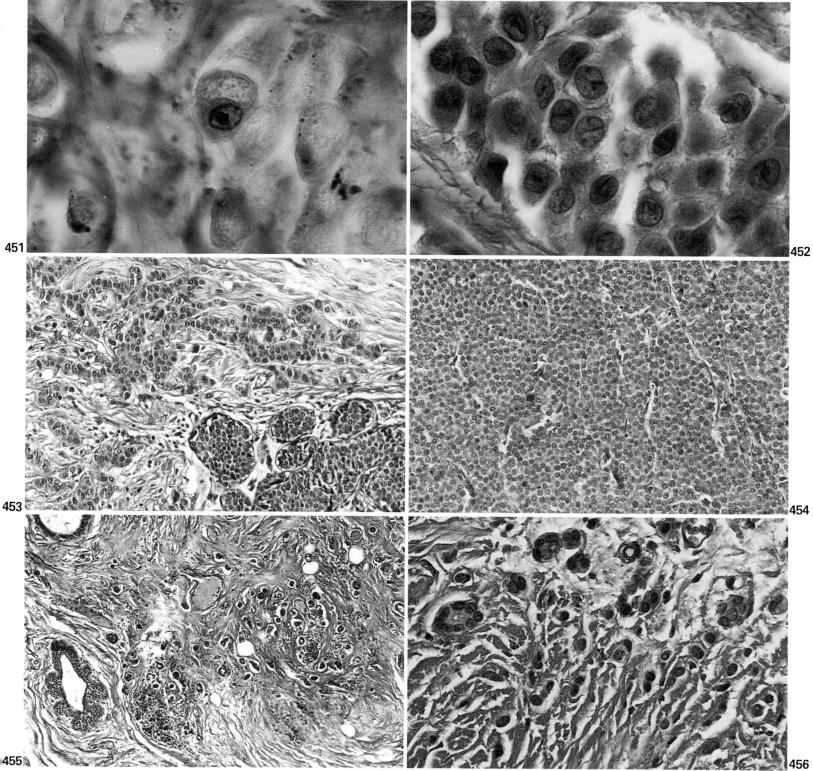

SIGNET RING CELL CARCINOMA

Carcinoma composed of cells which contain a cytoplasmic mucin-positive vacuole displacing the nucleus towards a pole. The histogenesis of the pure form of this carcinoma remains controversial: is it a variant of invasive lobular carcinoma or of mucinous carcinoma? Large foci of such cells can be found in various types of otherwise typical carcinomas (invasive ductal carcinoma, mucinous carcinoma, invasive ductal carcinoma, ductal carcinoma in situ). However, such a component is particularly frequent in ILC in which the intracellular vacuole ultrastructurally corresponds to an 'intracytoplasmic lumen' (space lined by microvilli and containing a central core of mucin). In other carcinomas, the mucin is most often packaged in round granules bounded by smooth membranes.

HISTIOCYTOID CARCINOMA

The term 'histiocytoid' only reflects the histiocytic appearance of carcinomatous cells, which have an abundant cytoplasm, either acidophile or microvacuolized. This term leads to confusion because it is used for a variant of lipid-secreting breast carcinoma (Van Bogaert). But unlike this carcinoma, the histiocytoid carcinoma is characterized by mucin-positive and lipid-negative reactions. Histogenesis of the pure form is controversial, either invasive lobular carcinoma or mucinous carcinoma. Foci of such cells can be observed in both these types of carcinoma. Recently, apocrine markers have been found in histiocytoid carcinoma (Eusebi).

457 HES ×64: *Alveolar type*
Alveolar grouping of tumour cells invading the smooth muscle bundles of the nipple (which allows to distinguish it here from a lobular carcinoma in situ). Most often, this variant is accompanied with a typical pattern.

458 HES ×160: 'Signet-ring cell' carcinoma.

459 HES ×64
460 EMA ×160
'Histiocytoid' cells with a large acidophile cytoplasm, which is strongly stained with EMA.

461 HES ×64
462 AB ×160
'Histiocytoid' cells with small nuclei and abundant cytoplasm that contains AB-positive vacuoles.

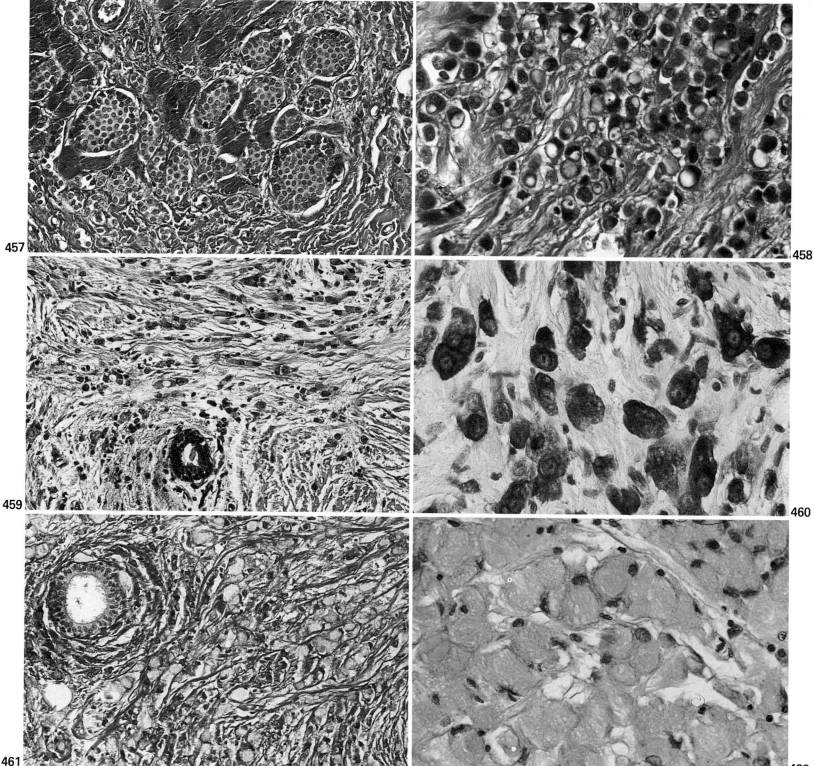

457

458

459

460

461

462

MUCINOUS CARCINOMA

Synonyms

Gelatinous carcinoma, colloid carcinoma.

Definition

'A carcinoma containing large amounts of extra-cellular epithelial mucus, sufficient to be visible macroscopically and recognizable microscopically surrounding and within tumour cells.'

Nosology

The pure form of mucinous carcinoma is easy to classify, but in the case of partial mucinous compo-nent, the carcinoma (mucinous, invasive ductal or mixed type) is not covered by most of the classifica-tions.

Clinical features

- Rare form: 2.5%
- Slow growth and better prognosis than invasive ductal carcinoma
- High mean age: 63 years.

Histological features

- Usually well-defined contours
- Frequent intraductal component
- A low cellularity should be a factor of better prognosis (factor independent of tumour size)
- Frequent argyrophil variant.

Differential diagnosis

Pseudo-mucinous carcinoma.

463 Macroscopy
Round and well-circumscribed nodule with shining, soft and sticky cut surface. Such a macroscopic pat-tern may also correspond to a fibroadenoma with myxoid stroma.

464 HES ×25
Low cellularity. Small clusters of cells with some tubule formation surrounded by mucin; some thin collagen fibres.

465 Mucicarmin ×25
Intraductal component with abundant mucin within the lumen.

466 HES ×25
IDC with partial mucinous component (<25%).

467 Grandi alcian blue ×64
(A combined alcian blue and Grimelius staining technique.) All tumour cells contain argyrophil cytoplasmic granules. Argyrophil cells are par-ticularly frequent in mucinous carcinomas.

468 HES ×25
Pseudomucinous carcinoma. The interstitial sub-stance corresponds to oedema dissociating collagen fibres. Mucin stainings are negative.

MEDULLARY CARCINOMA

Definition

'A well-circumscribed carcinoma composed of poorly differentiated cells with scant stroma and prominent lymphoid infiltration. The tumour cells are large with vesicular nuclei, prominent nucleoli and indistinct cytoplasmic outlines. Sheets and broad anastomosing cords without gland-like struc-tures are the usual growth form. Tumour borders should be histologically blunt and ''pushing'', not insinuating and tentacular.'

Nosology

Some authors have expressed a doubt about the favourable prognosis and the specific morphologic definition of the lesion as a distinct clinicopathologic entity. In spite of the precise criteria defined by Ridolfi (1977), the diagnosis remains difficult and it would be interesting to control the reproducibility of such a diagnosis.

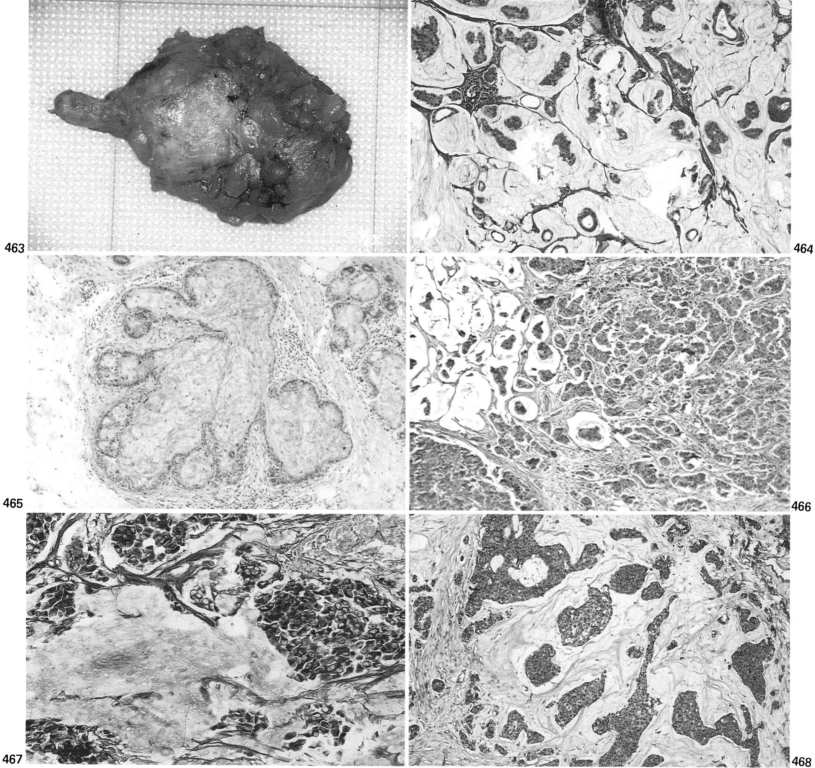

463
464
465
466
467
468

Clinical features

- Rare form: 1 to 6% according to series.
- Round and mobile tumour which mimics fibro-adenoma.
- Better prognosis than IDC.

Histological features

Have been detailed by Ridolfi (1977). See table below of criteria borrowed from the author:

Typical medullary (All of the following features)	Atypical medullary (Features of typical medullary but with any of the following)	Nonmedullary infiltrating duct carcinoma
• predominantly syncytial growth pattern (>75%)	• predominantly syncytial growth pattern (>75%)	• syncytial growth pattern <75% and/or presence of three or more other atypical features
• microscopically completely circumscribed	• areas of tumour margins show focal or prominent infiltration	
• no intraductal component	• intraductal carcinoma present or prominent	
• moderate to marked diffuse mononuclear stromal infiltrate	• mild or negligible mononuclear infiltrate or infiltrate at margins only	
• nuclear grade 1 or 2	• nuclear grade 3	
• absence of microglandular features	• presence of microglandular features	

Note: Squamous, cartilaginous, or spindle-cell metaplasia and areas of papillary differentiation did not influence carcinoma subclassification.

The cell atypia are marked for nuclear grade 1, moderate for grade 2, slight for grade 3 (Black, 1957).

Nevertheless the authors found in the course of their study that certain criteria which exclude a lesion from the medullary carcinoma category did not affect survival:

- an intraductal component; consequently, the authors have redistributed these cases in the typical medullary group
- a focal microglandular differentiation or focal infiltration at the periphery of an otherwise typical medullary carcinoma. This should not exclude the diagnosis of medullary carcinoma.

Differential diagnosis

With an invasive ductal carcinoma which may be circumscribed with inflammatory stroma but where the growth pattern is trabecular (not syncytial) and the fibrous stroma more abundant.

469 Mammography
Round tumour with well-defined contours without signs of malignancy.

470 Macroscopy
Round, well-circumscribed, soft tumour, but with suspicious central necrotic area.

471 HES ×10
'Pushing'-type tumour borders with a fibrous pseudocapsule.

472 HES ×160
Syncytial growth: broad anastomosing bands of tumour cells with indistinct borders 'embryonal carcinoma-like'. This syncytial-type pattern should constitute 75% or more of the growth pattern for a tumour to be included in the medullary category. It must be distinguished from trabecular growth characterized by narrow cords of cells with distinct cell borders and inconspicuous or absent inter-anastomosing areas.

473 HES ×160
Marked nuclear pleomorphism with malignant giant cells.

474 HES ×25
Marked central necrosis surrounded by syncytial-like bands of tumour cells.

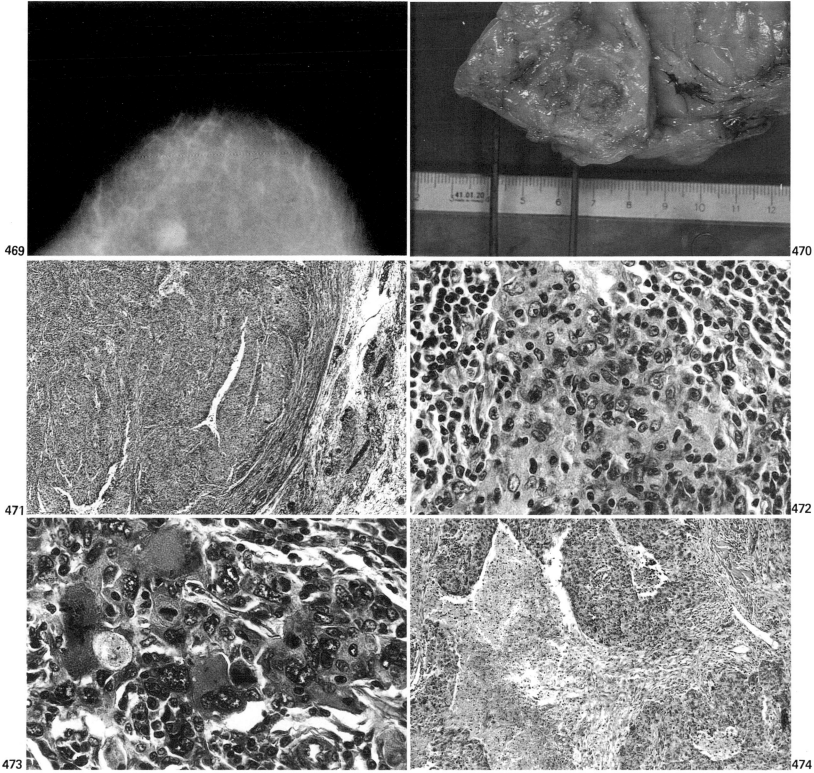

469

470

471

472

473

474

PAPILLARY CARCINOMA

Definition

'A rare carcinoma whose invasive pattern is predominantly in the form of papillary structures.' The papillary architecture is usually displayed in the metastases and intraductal component.

Nosology

This term has to be distinguished from invasive ductal carcinoma which contain a papillary intraductal component. Fisher includes in the category, carcinomas with some solid-appearing areas.

Clinical features

- Rare form (2%),
- Favourable prognosis,
- Post-menopausal age.

Histological features

- Usually well-defined contours,
- Marked papillary intraductal component,
- Frequent microcalcifications,
- Architectural pattern: predominantly papillary with some cribriform, tubular or solid areas,
- Cells: common or apocrine type.

Differential diagnosis

- invasive ductal carcinoma with a papillary intraductal component,
- pseudopapillary lymphatic invasion (see page 168).

475 HES ×25 ⎫
476 HES ×64 ⎭
Area of invasive papillary carcinoma: some papillae contain conspicuous stroma stalks, others are filiform or finger-like.

477 HES ×25
Area of adenomatoid configuration.

478 HES ×25
Epithelial projections with inconspicuous supporting stalks: reticular pattern.

479 HES ×64
Solid-appearing area.

480 HES ×64
Papillary intraductal component with microcalcifications.

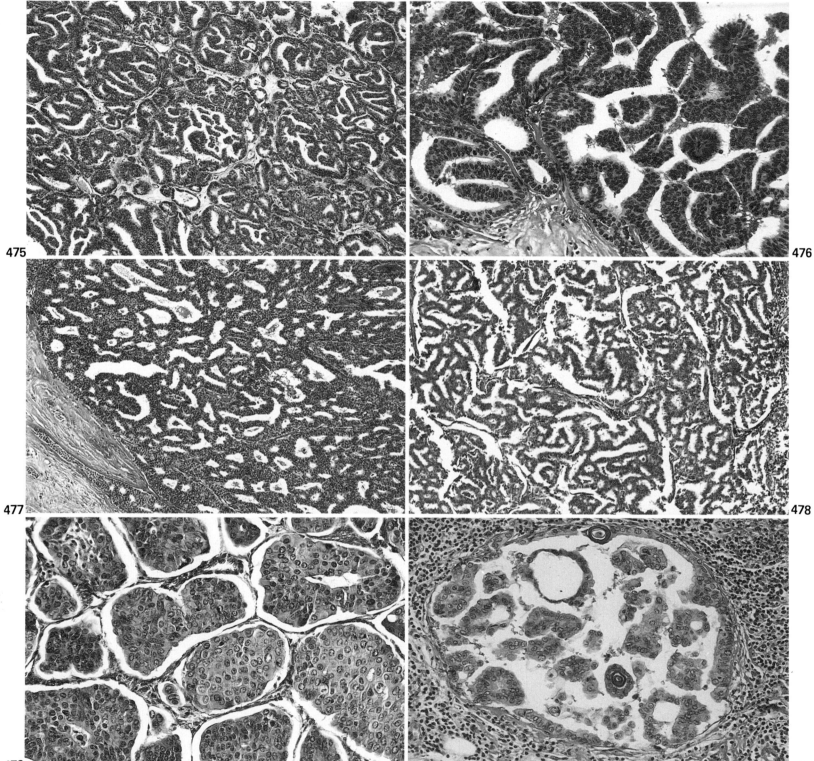

TUBULAR CARCINOMA

Synonyms

'Well-differentiated' or 'orderly' carcinoma.

Definition

'A highly differentiated invasive carcinoma whose cells are regular and arranged in well-defined tubules typically one layer thick and surrounded by an abundant fibrous stroma.'

Nosology

This type includes the pure type and for some authors the mixed type (tubular component more than 75%).

Clinical features

- Rare form with favourable prognosis (2 to 10%).
- Frequent multicentricity and bilaterality.

Histological features

- Stellate small-sized carcinoma.
- Intraductal component (70% of cases).
- Early tubular carcinoma in the centre of a radial scar (see Chapter 2, page 48).

Differential diagnosis

- with adenosis either sclerosing or microglandular (see Chapter 2, pages 32 and 36),
- with invasive ductal carcinoma (here tubular structures are irregular with atypical and multi-layered epithelium).

481   Mammography
Stellate tumour.

482   HES ×10
Tubular carcinoma (6mm) with spicules and infiltration into the surrounding fat.

483   HES ×64
Tubules with a single cell layer without cytonuclear atypia, nor mitosis. Appearance of open tubular structures with 'angulated' contours.

484   HES ×160
Spur-like distorted tubule.

485   HES ×160
Open tubules lined by epithelial cells with apocrine snouts.

486   HES ×25
Angulated tubules with trabecular bars partitioning occasional lumina.

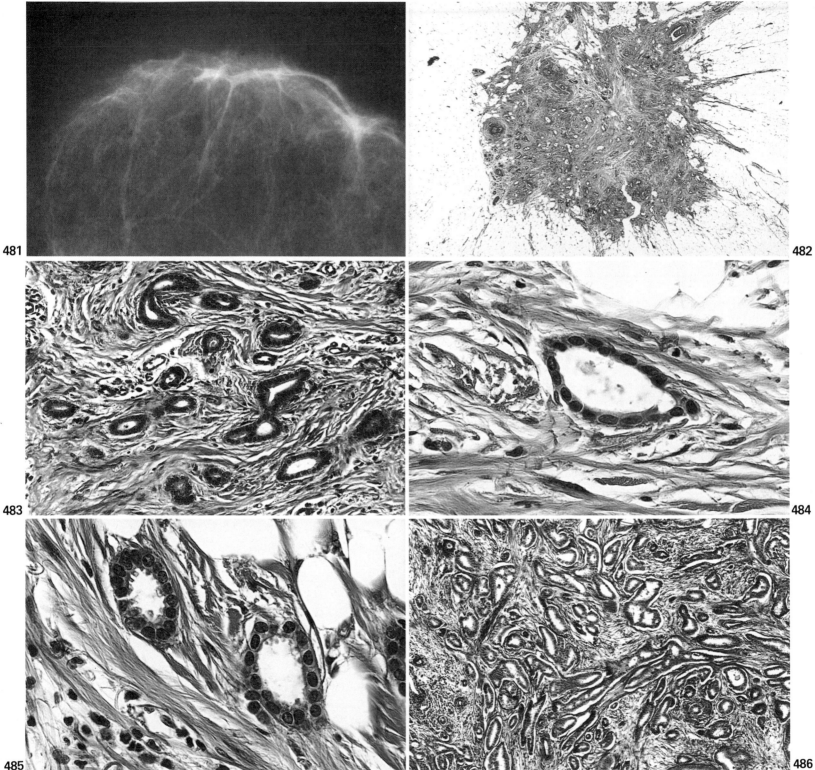

ADENOID CYSTIC CARCINOMA

Synonym

Adenocystic carcinoma, cylindroma.

Terminology

The denomination 'cylindroma' originates from the stromal cores or 'cylinders' within the nests of tumour cells, responsible for the cribriform pattern.

Definition

'An invasive carcinoma having a characteristic cribriform appearance' comparable to the same type of tumour in the salivary glands.

Histogenesis

The origin of the proliferative cells is controversial: ductal and/or myoepithelial, or pluripotential stem cell capable, as in the salivary gland, of differentiation into ductal, myoepithelial and acinar cells.

Clinical features

- rare form with favourable prognosis (<1%).
- exceptional lymph node metastases.

Histological features

| Two types of cells |
| Two types of mucins |
| Two types of markers |

Two populations of cells

- small basaloid cells arranged according to several growth patterns (solid, cribriform or tubular) which frequently are mixed although any one may predominate.
- epithelial cells arranged around true glandular lumina.

Mucins

One in the pseudocysts, stained with AB, the other in the true glandular lumina stained with PAS.

Immunohistochemical markers

Coexpression of keratin and vimentin filaments and positivity of a few cells with S100 protein.

Differential diagnosis

With a ductal carcinoma in situ and an invasive ductal carcinoma, with cribriform pattern where the glandular spaces are more rigid and regular with a polarity of epithelial cells around lumina.

487 HES ×25
488 PAS ×160
'Solid' pattern: solid masses rarely punctuated with a few hyaline 'cylinders' strongly stained with PAS.

489 HES ×25
'Cribriform' pattern: pseudocysts containing a mucoid material. This extracellular matrix material is synthesized by the tumour cells and corresponds to the accumulation of basement membrane material, proteoglycans and sometimes collagen.

490 HES ×64
'Tubular' pattern: tubule-like structures with a lumen lined by few rows (1 to 3) of haphazardly orientated basaloid cells.

491 HES ×64
492 Cytok ×64
Cribriform mass with biphasic cellular population: small glandular lumina are well visible between pseudocysts. These glands are strongly stained with cytokeratin.

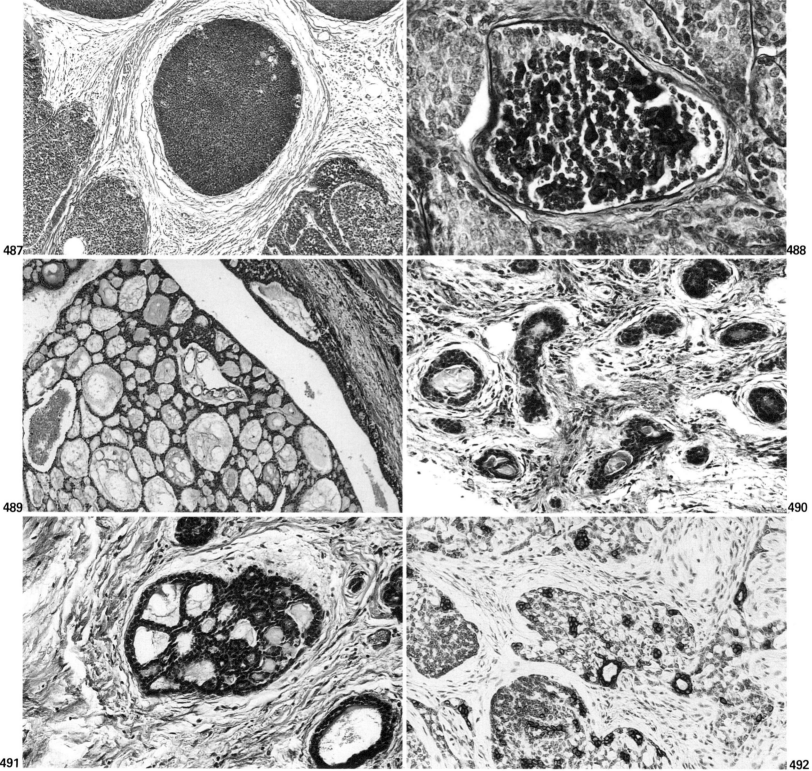

APOCRINE CARCINOMA

Synonyms

Oncocytic carcinoma, sweat gland carcinoma, pink-cell carcinoma.

Definition

'A carcinoma composed predominantly of cells with abundant eosinophilic cytoplasm reminiscent of metaplastic apocrine cells.'

Nosology

Foci of apocrine tumour cells may be seen in other types of mammary carcinoma but the pure (or predominant) form only accounts for this category. However, two points must be underlined, no account of the apocrine component has been stated precisely and the diagnostic criteria are subjective (that explains the variable frequency of this carcinoma: less than 1% to 14%). Fisher (1975) denies the existence of a pure form of apocrine carcinoma.

- Frequency of apocrine DCIS (papillary or cribriform pattern)
- Apocrine cells:
  (i) copious granular and acidophilic cytoplasm
  (ii) presence of PAS-positive diastase-resistant apical granules and of apical snouts
  (iii) large round nuclei with a prominent nucleolus
- Immunohistochemical marker of apocrine differentiation: GCDFP-15 protein, a protein present in apocrine epithelium and in the fluid of tension cysts.

493 HES ×25 ⎫
494 HES ×64 ⎬
195 HES ×160 ⎭
Apocrine carcinoma with solid pattern and area of necrosis.

496 HES ×64 ⎫
497 D-PAS ×160 ⎬
498 D-PAS ×400 ⎭
Apocrine carcinoma with papillary pattern. PAS-positive diastase-resistant apical granules.

CARCINOMA WITH METAPLASIA

Definition

Invasive ductal carcinoma with various types of metaplastic alterations (squamous, spindle-cell, cartilaginous, osseous or mixed type).

Terminology – Nosology

The term 'carcinosarcoma' refers to:
- a mixed histological pattern of carcinoma and sarcoma, without taking into account pathogenesis,
- a true carcinosarcoma, that is, a collision between two distinct proliferations, the one carcinomatous originating from the epithelial component, the other sarcomatous originating from the mesenchymal component. Carcinosarcomas arising in a fibroadenoma or in a phyllodes tumour are likely to be the only true ones.

Currently, it is accepted by most authors that the sarcomatous appearance arises by direct metaplasia of the carcinomatous cells. These metaplastic cells can produce collagen, mature or immature osseous or cartilaginous material.

Metaplasia may be of:

- Spindle-cell type.
- Squamous type, wholly or partly. This group includes the 'spindle-cell carcinoma' equivalent in the breast to the well-recognized entity in the larynx, oral cavity, oesophagus and skin.
- Cartilaginous and osseous type: the cartilaginous and osseous areas having a benign or malignant appearance. These tumours look like salivary gland tumours and are termed by some authors 'malignant mixed tumours'. They are very frequent in dogs.

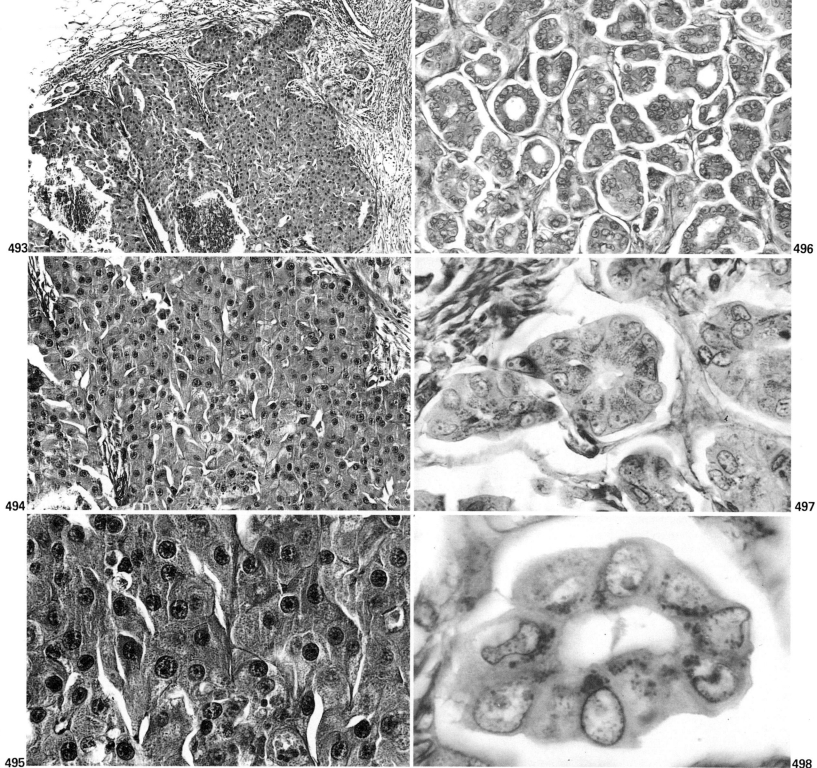

Immunohistochemical features

- cytokeratin and/or EMA
  - (i) always positive in epithelial cells
  - (ii) negative or positive in a variable number of spindle cells.
- vimentin
  - (i) negative in epithelial cells
  - (ii) positive in a varying number of spindle cells, rarely totally negative.
- possible coexpression of vimentin and cytokeratin in a few spindle cells.

Clinical and histological features

Vary according to the type of metaplastic carcinoma (see below).

Differential diagnosis

With an invasive ductal carcinoma with anaplastic pattern.

CARCINOMA WITH SPINDLE-CELL METAPLASIA

Definition

IDC with pseudosarcomatous spindle-cell metaplasia

Clinical features

- Rare form.
- Large-sized tumour.
- Rare lymph node metastases.
- Prognosis depends on the amount of sarcomatous component.

Histological features

- Appearance of biphasic tumour with an epithelial component and a sarcomatous-like component (10 to 90%) which may be of:
  - fibrosarcomatous type
  - malignant histiocytofibroma type
  - anaplastic type with malignant or osteoclast-like giant cells.
- Axillary nodal metastases are purely epithelial as opposed to distant metastases, often mixed.

499 Cytok ×10
500 Cytok ×160
501 Vim ×160

Biphasic tumour with predominant carcinomatous component and areas of spindle-cell metaplasia (the latter showing cytokeratin-positive cells and vimentin-positive cells).

502 HES ×25
503 HES ×64
504 Cytok ×64

Biphasic tumour: small carcinomatous component and predominance of metaplastic areas with malignant cytokeratin-negative giant cells.

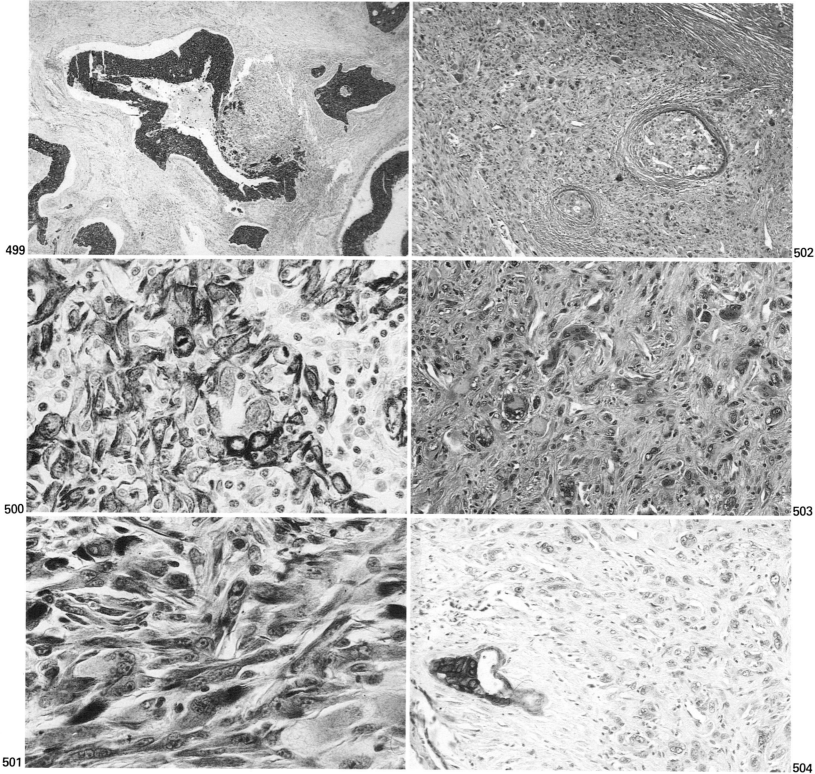

CARCINOMA WITH SQUAMOUS METAPLASIA

IDC with partial squamous metaplasia

This metaplasia may occur in all histologic types of carcinoma (3.7%) without changing the prognosis (Fisher, 1975).

Pure squamous cell carcinoma

It is unclear if such a carcinoma constitutes a distinct entity which has to be separated from metaplastic carcinomas. The origin is debated: ductal origin with squamous metaplasia or epidermal or dermoid cyst origin (the latter because of frequent cystic appearances observed in this cancer). Such a diagnosis implies:

- absence of glandular features (to be distinguished from a mucoepidermoid carcinoma)
- exclusion of a tumour of cutaneous origin (absence of anatomic relationship with the epidermis)
- exclusion of a metastasis of squamous carcinoma.

Spindle-cell carcinoma

Synonyms

Squamous spindle-cell carcinoma, sarcomatoid squamous carcinoma, pseudosarcomatous carcinoma, pleomorphic carcinoma.

Clinical features

- The same prognosis as invasive ductal carcinoma.
- Larger tumour.
- Fewer lymph node metastases.

Histological features

> - **Biphasic tumour with a squamous component and a spindle-cell component.**
> - **Sometimes stromal reaction with osteoclast-like giant cells.**

505 HES ×25
IDC with partial squamous metaplasia, visible glands and fibroblastic stroma.

506 HES ×64
Pure squamous carcinoma. The squamous differentiation is obvious.

507 HES ×64 ⎱
508 HES ×160 ⎰
Spindle-cell carcinoma consisting of epithelial nests with obvious squamous differentiation and sarcomatoid spindle-cell areas.

509 HES ×64 ⎱
510 Cytok ×64 ⎰
Spindle-cell carcinoma with many cytokeratin-positive cells.

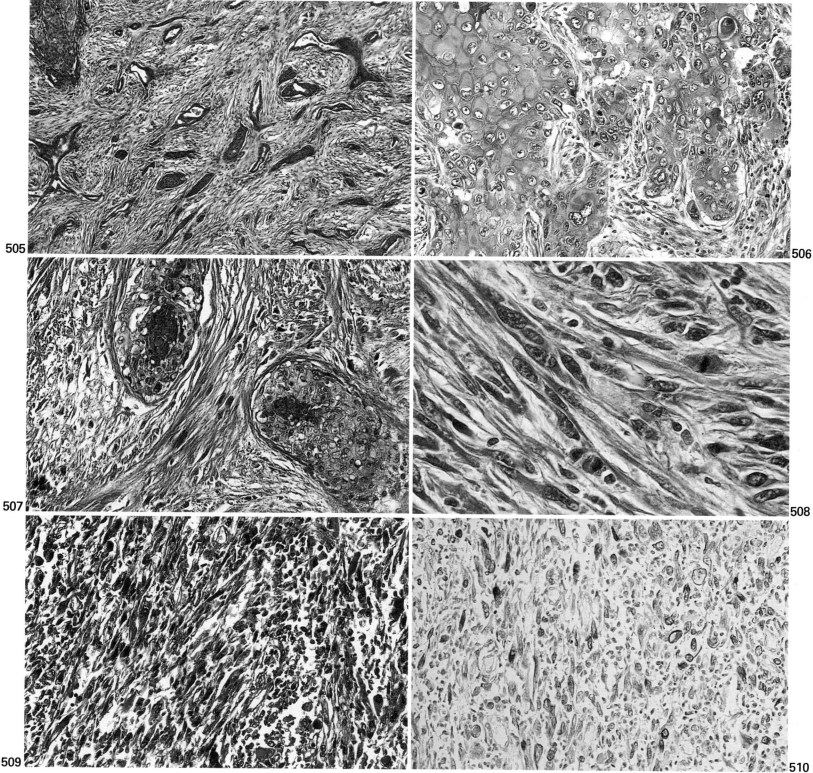

Differential diagnosis

With anaplastic pattern of invasive carcinoma.

511 HES ×64 ⎫
512 Cytok ×64 ⎭
Carcinoma with anaplastic appearance, but the carcinomatous nature is obvious after cytokeratin staining: all cells are strongly positive.

513 HES ×160 ⎫
514 Cytok ×160 ⎭
Anaplastic carcinoma with giant cells and inflammatory stroma. The carcinomatous nature is confirmed by the strong cytokeratin positivity of all cells.

515 HES ×64 ⎫
516 EMA ×160 ⎭
Anaplastic proliferation, the carcinomatous or sarcomatous nature of which is difficult to assess. A small cluster of cells shows an EMA positivity arguing for a carcinoma.

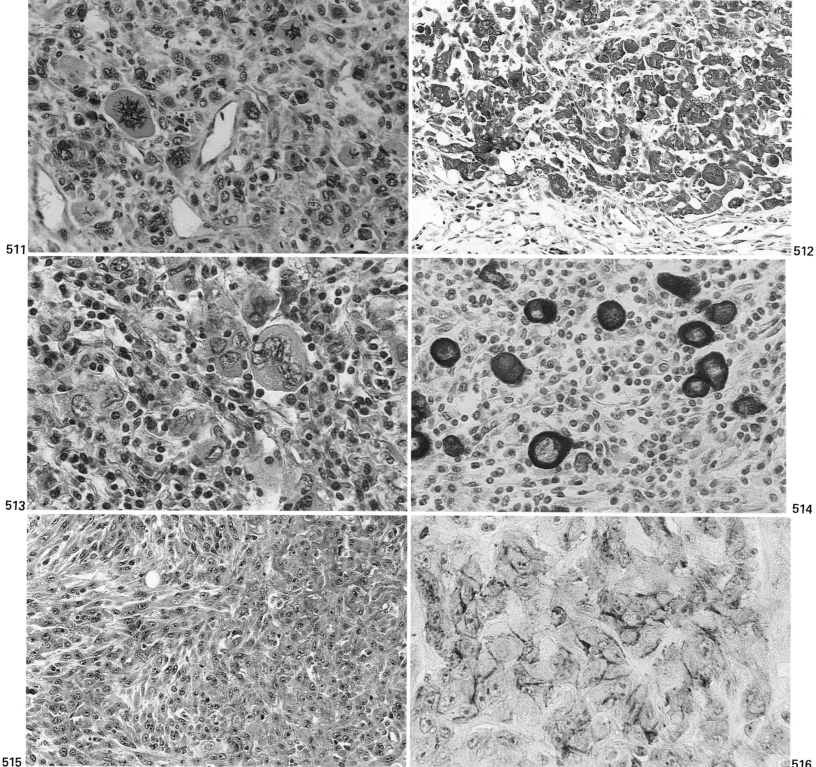

OTHER INVASIVE CARCINOMAS

BREAST CARCINOMA WITH OSTEOCLAST-LIKE GIANT CELLS

Definition

Invasive carcinoma of all histologic types (ductal, lobular or metaplastic carcinoma), with osteoclast-like giant cells.

Genesis

Giant cells have a stromal origin and arise from fusion of mononuclear stromal histiocytes. Their presence could be induced by a factor produced by carcinomatous cells. The same factor might induce hypervascularity (although not proved).

Clinical features

- Premenopausal age of the patients
- Prognosis comparable with an invasive breast cancer of same histological type

Histopathological features

- Osteoclast-like giant cells
  (i) are found in the stroma and within glandular lumina of the tumour,
  (ii) are also present in nodal or distant metastases,
- The tumour stroma contains an increased vascularity, hemorrhages and hemosiderin deposits.

Immunohistochemical features

---
of giant cells:
- **epithelial markers negative**
- **histiocytic markers usually negative**
- **leucocyte common antigen and vimentin positive.**

Note
- The often benign mammographic appearance of the tumour due to well-circumscribed contours,
- A characteristic gross feature: reddish-brown colour of the tumour.

517 HES ×25
Papillary carcinoma with 'cart-wheel' pattern. Giant cells are found in the stroma and within the epithelial component.

518 HES ×64
A giant cell in close proximity with an area of hemorrhage; opening of ductal lumen in the stroma.

519 HES ×160
A giant cell within a gland lumen.

520 HES ×160
Presence within a gland lumen of giant cells and mononuclear precursors.

521 HES ×64
Numerous giant cells in IDC.

522 Cytok ×160
Strong positivity of epithelial cells and negativity of giant cells.

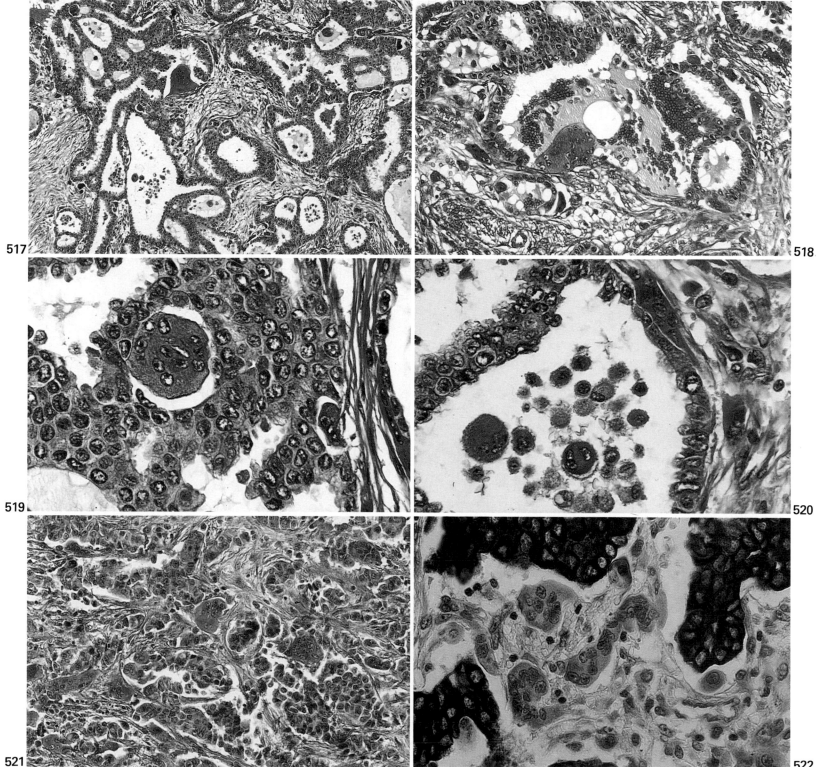

SECRETORY (JUVENILE) CARCINOMA

'A carcinoma with pale-staining cells showing prominent secretory activity of the type seen in pregnancy and lactation. PAS-positive material is present in the cytoplasm and in acinar-like spaces.'

Clinical features

- Is found more frequently in children.
- Has a favourable prognosis.

Histological features

- Large amounts of intra- and extra-cellular mucin.
- Growth patterns: tubular, acinar, cribriform, solid.
- Cells: abundant, clear or vacuolized cytoplasm.

Differential diagnosis

- with a lipid-secreting carcinoma (in which the mucin stainings are negative)
  with other mucin-secreting carcinomas (signet-ring cell, histiocytoid, mucinous carcinomas): according to localization and amount of mucin.

523 AB ×64
524 AB ×160
Solid pattern with abundant intra- and extracellular secretory material, strongly stained with alcian blue.

GLYCOGEN-RICH CLEAR-CELL CARCINOMA

Tumour composed exclusively or predominantly of clear cells with abundant glycogen. Similar areas are frequently found in invasive ductal carcinoma or ductal carcinoma in situ. Prognosis of the pure form appears almost similar to that of invasive ductal carcinoma-NOS.

525 PAS ×64
526 D-PAS ×64
Solid pattern with infiltration of adipose tissue. The cytoplasm of cells is filled with glycogen stained by PAS and appears clear after diastasic digestion.

LIPID-SECRETING CARCINOMA

Carcinoma composed of cells with foamy cytoplasm and large amounts of lipids (similar to cells of histiocytoid carcinoma but without intracytoplasmic mucin). Fisher does not agree with this entity because he has observed in one third of breast cancers of any histologic type a moderate or marked lipid secretion.

527 HES ×64
528 PAS ×160
The majority of cells have a finely vacuolated cytoplasm. Clear vacuoles contain lipids but not mucin (PAS negative).

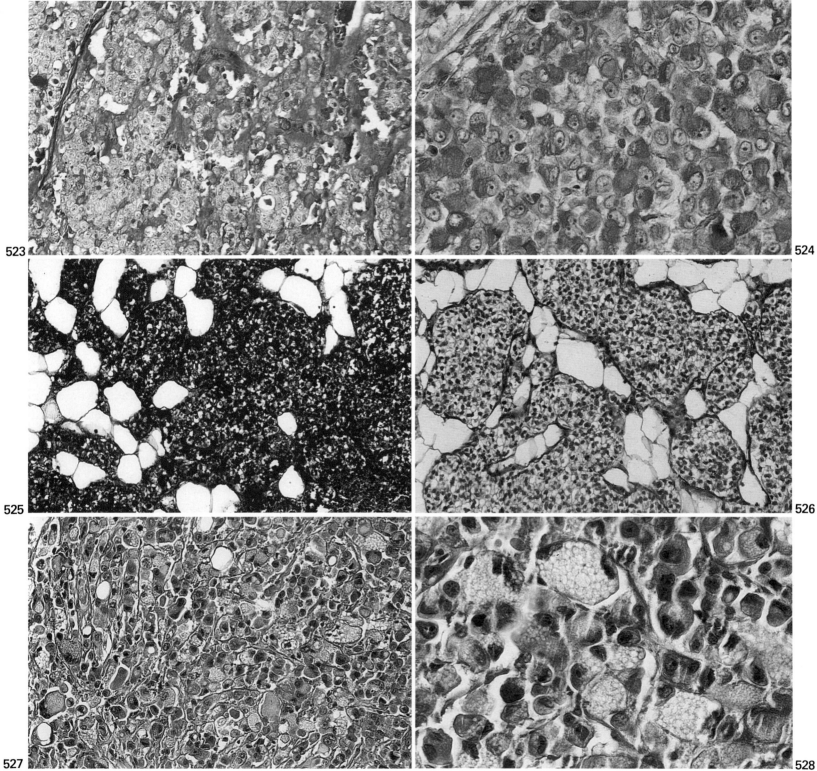

7.3 PAGET'S DISEASE OF THE NIPPLE

Definition
'A lesion in which large pale-staining cells are present within the epidermis of the nipple.'

Nosology
It is classified either in the associated carcinoma (ductal carcinoma in situ or invasive ductal carcinoma), or in an independent group.

Histogenesis
Two theories:
- an 'epidermotropic' cancer, i.e. migration of Paget cells towards the nipple epidermis from an underlying breast carcinoma,
- carcinoma in situ of intraepidermal origin. Paget cells would originate from malignant change either of keratinocytes (directly or after glandular metaplasia) or of intraepidermal heterotopic glandular cells.

> Paget's disease might be 'part of the general phenomenon of multicentricity in breast cancer' (spread or local genesis).

Clinical features
- incidence: 2% of breast cancers
- mean age: 54 years
- nipple lesion: discharge, reddening, erosion evolving slowly (to be distinguished from nipple adenoma or dermatitis)
- sometimes underlying tumour or foci of microcalcifications.

Histopathological features

> - Rarely confined to the epidermis, most often associated with an underlying carcinoma (ductal carcinoma in situ or invasive ductal carcinoma).
> - Infiltration of the epidermis by Paget cells either single or in nests or in glands, without infiltration of the dermis. Cells may contain mucin.
> - Frequent involvement of milk sinuses.

Differential diagnosis
- with a direct invasion of the skin by a mammary carcinoma
- with a superficial spreading melanoma (Paget cells can contain melanin granules).

529 HES ×64
Paget cells scattered through the epidermis.

530 HES ×64
Paget cells forming solid nests or glands.

531 HES ×160
Melanin granules in a few Paget cells.

532 HES ×25
Paget cells in the ductal epithelium as the duct terminates in the nipple epidermis.

533 Cytok ×64
534 EMA ×64
Paget cells are weakly positive with cytokeratin staining while squamous cells are strongly positive. Conversely, Paget cells are strongly positive with EMA staining as is the ductal epithelium while squamous cells are negative or very weakly positive. For some authors, this staining pattern supports the hypothesis that Paget cells are malignant ductal cells.

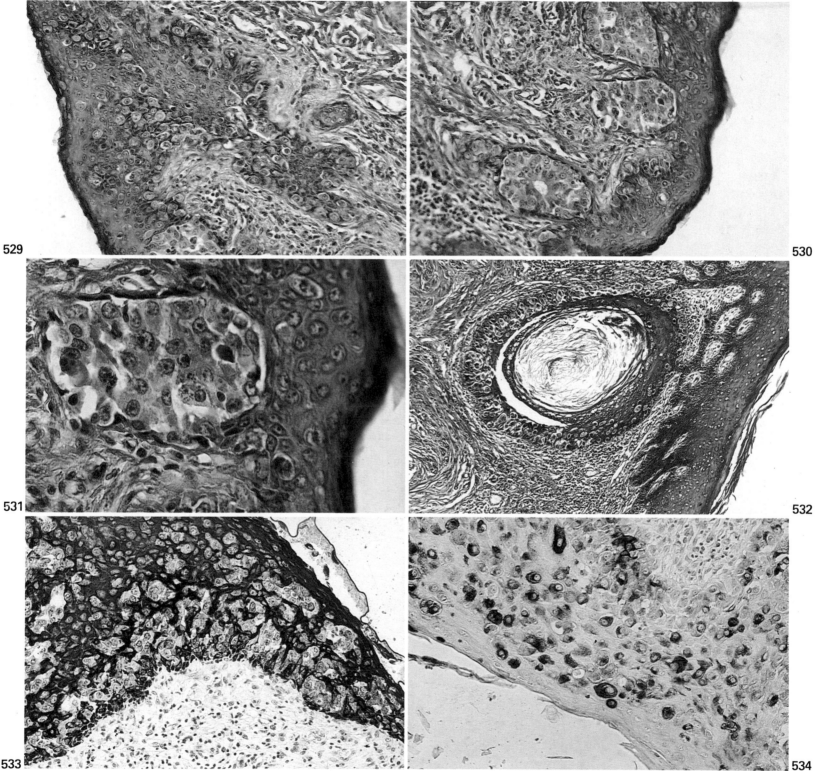

529

530

531

532

533

534

7.4 COMBINATIONS OF HISTOLOGICAL TYPES IN THE SAME TUMOUR MASS

These combinations are frequent and difficult to classify. According to the WHO, 'if a component is a minor one only, the tumour should be classified by the predominant pattern. Extensive mixtures, however, require multiple diagnoses'. These indications only deal with the quantitative and not qualitative features of the neoplastic components and undervalue the mixtures.

Fisher resolves the problem by listing every morphological feature of a tumour and by designating the tumour as a pure tumour or as combinations of tumour types.

Here are two examples of a mixture of invasive ductal carcinoma and invasive lobular carcinoma, in which the invasive lobular carcinoma component is very small but cannot be denied; it is associated with lobular carcinoma in situ in one of the cases.

Case 1 combination of invasive ductal carcinoma and ILC

535 HES ×25
Invasive ductal carcinoma (with marked intraductal component not visible here).

536 HES ×25
Mixture in the same ducts of intraductal component and lobular carcinoma in situ.

537 HES ×64
Near lobular carcinoma in situ, single or in-file cells, typical of ILC, quite different from predominant invasive ductal carcinoma component.

Case 2 combination of invasive ductal carcinoma and ILC

538 HES ×64
Two cell components with very different growth patterns and cytological appearance, one invasive ductal carcinoma type, the other ILC type.

539 HES ×160
Invasive ductal carcinoma trabeculae.

540 HES ×160
Difference between the two cell components is obvious.

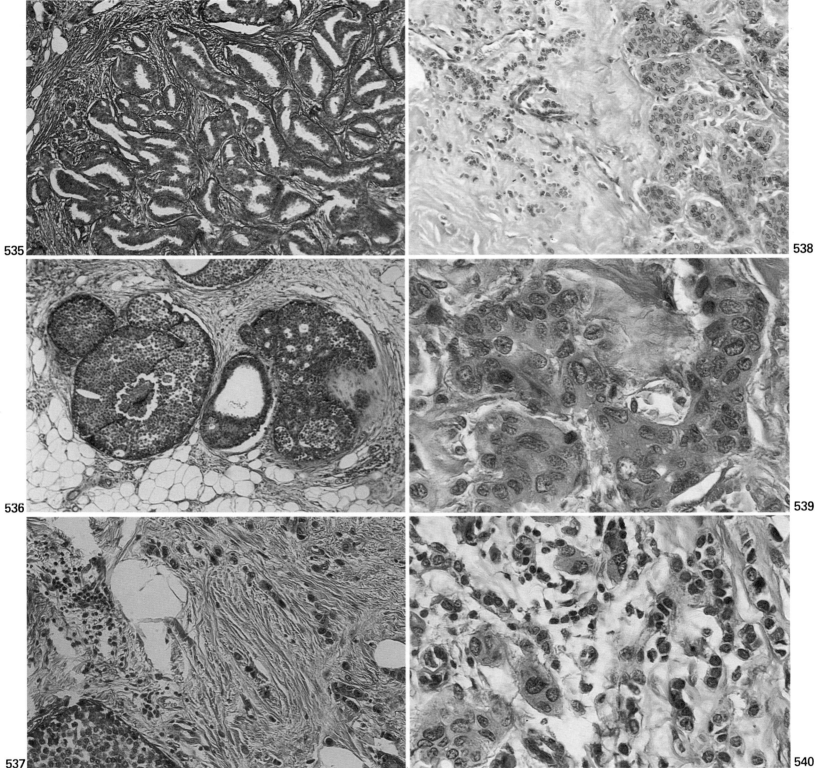

535

536

537

538

539

540

References
Chap. 7 – Carcinomas

Trojani, M. *et al.* (1984) types histologiques de 876 cancers du sein selon l'O.M.S. *Bull. Cancer* (Paris), **71**, 65.

LOBULAR CARCINOMA IN SITU

Eusebi, V. *et al.* (1984) Apocrine differentiation in lobular carcinoma of the breast. *Hum. Pathol.*, **15**, 134.

Foote, F.W. *et al.* (1941) Lobular carcinoma in situ. *Am. J. Pathol.*, **17**, 491.

Frykberg, E.R. *et al.* (1987) Lobular carcinoma in situ of the breast. *Surg. Gynecol. Obstet.*, **164**, 285.

Haagensen, C.D. *et al.* (1978) Lobular neoplasia (socalled lobular carcinoma in situ) of the breast. *Cancer*, **42**, 737.

Haagensen, C.D. *et al.* (1983) Coexisting lobular neoplasia and carcinoma of the breast. *Cancer*, **51**, 1468.

Page, D.L. *et al.* (1985) Atypical hyperplastic lesions of the female breast. *Cancer*, **55**, 2698.

Rosen, P.P. *et al.* (1978) Lobular carcinoma in situ of the breast. Detailed analysis of 99 patients with average follow-up of 24 years. *Am. J. Surg. Pathol.*, **2**, 225.

Rosen, P.P. *et al.* (1980) Coexisting lobular carcinoma in situ and intraductal carcinoma in a single lobular-duct unit. *Am. J. Surg. Pathol.*, **4**, 241.

Rosen, P.P. *et al.* (1981) Lobular carcinoma in situ. Preliminary results of treatment by ipsilateral mastectomy and contralateral breast biopsy. *Cancer*, **47**, 813.

Webber, B.L. *et al.* (1981) Risk of subsequent contralateral breast carcinoma in a population of patients with in situ breast carcinoma. *Cancer*, **47**, 2928.

DUCTAL CARCINOMA IN SITU

Ashikari, R. *et al.* (1971) Intraductal carcinoma of the breast. *Cancer*, **28**, 1182.

Betsill, W.L. *et al.* (1978) Intraductal carcinoma: long-term follow-up after treatment by biopsy alone. *J.A.M.A.*, **239**, 1863.

Contesso, G. *et al.* (1977) Les facteurs anatomopathologiques du pronostic des cancers du sein. *Bull. Cancer*, **64**, 525.

Cowen, P.N. *et al.* (1984) The significance of intraduct appearances in breast cancer. *Clin. Oncol.*, **10**, 67

Fentiman, I.S. *et al.* (1986) In situ ductal carcinoma of the breast: implications of disease pattern and treatment. *Eur. J. Surg. Oncol.*, **12**, 261.

Fisher, E.R. *et al.* (1986) Pathologic findings from the National Surgical Adjuvant Breast Project (Protocol 6): I. Intraductal carcinoma (D.C.I.S.). *Cancer*, **57**, 197.

Lagios, M.D. *et al.* (1982) Duct carcinoma in situ. *Cancer*, **50**, 1309.

Page, D.L. *et al.* (1982) Intraductal carcinoma of the breast: follow-up after biopsy only. *Cancer*, **49**, 751.

Page, D.L. *et al.* (1985) Atypical hyperplastic lesions of the female breast. *Cancer*, **55**, 2698.

Rosen, P.P. *et al.* (1984) Cystic hypersecretory duct carcinoma of the breast. *Am. J. Surg. Pathol.*, **8**, 31.

Rosner, D. *et al.* (1980) Non invasive breast carcinoma. *Ann. Surg.*, **192**, 139.

INVASIVE DUCTAL CARCINOMA

Contours

Lane, N. *et al.* (1961) Clinicopathologic analysis of the surgical curability of breast cancers. *Ann. Surg.*, **153**, 483.

Silverberg, S.G. *et al.* (1971) Prognostic significance of tumor margins in mammary carcinoma. *Arch. Surg.*, **102**, 450.

Histological grading

Bloom, H.J.G. and Richardson, W.W. (1957) Histological grading and prognosis in breast cancer. *Br. J. Cancer*, **11**, 359.

Stenkvist, B. *et al.* (1979) Analysis of reproducibility of subjective grading systems for breast carcinoma. *J. Clin. Pathol.*, **32**, 979.

Stenkvist, B. *et al.* (1983) Histopathological systems of breast cancer classification. *J. Clin. Pathol.*, **36**, 392.

Stroma

Bogomoletz, W.V. (1986) Elastosis in breast cancer. *Pathology Annual.* Appleton-Century-Crofts, Norwalk, Connecticut, **21**, 347.

Fisher, E.R. *et al.* (1983) Types of tumor lymphoid response and sinus histiocytosis. *Arch. Pathol. Lab. Med.*, **107**, 222.

Fisher, E.R. *et al.* (1983) Scar cancers. *Breast Cancer Res. Treat.*, **3**, 39.

Rasmussen, B.B. *et al.* (1985) Elastosis in relation to prognosis in primary breast carcinoma. *Cancer Res.*, **45**, 1428.

Ross, M.J. *et al.* (1985) Sarcoidosis of the breast. *Hum. Pathol.*, **16**, 185.

ARGYROPHILIC CELLS IN CARCINOMA

Azzopardi, J.G. *et al.* (1982) 'Carcinoid' tumours of the breast: the morphological spectrum of argyrophil carcinomas. *Histopathology*, **6**, 549.

Bussolati, G. *et al.* (1987) Endocrine markers in argyrophilic carcinomas of the breast. *Am. J. Surg. Pathol.*, **11**, 248.

Fetissof, F. *et al.* (1983) Argyrophilic cells in mammary carcinoma. *Hum. Pathol.*, **14**, 127.

Forouhar, F.A. (1983) Morphologic study of carcinoid-like tumors and their relation to true carcinoids, using tumors of the breast as a model. *Tumori*, **69**, 171.

Partanen, S. *et al.* (1981) Argyrophilic cells in carcinoma of the female breast. *Virchows Arch* (Pathol. Anat.), **391**, 45.

Toyoshima, S. (1983) Mammary carcinoma with argyrophil cells. *Cancer*, **52**, 2129.

MUCUS AND GLYCOGEN

Battifora, H. *et al.* (1975) Intracytoplasmic lumina in breast carcinoma. *Arch. Pathol.*, **99**, 614.

Harris, M. *et al.* (1978) Mucin-producing carcinomas of the breast. *Histopathology*, **2**, 177.

Spriggs, A.I. *et al.* (1975) Intracellular mucous inclusions, a feature of malignant cells in effusions in the serous cavities, particularly due to carcinoma of the breast. *J. Clin. Pathol.*, **28**, 929.

IMMUNOHISTOCHEMISTRY: EPITHELIAL MARKERS

Berry, N. *et al.* (1985) The prognostic value of the monoclonal antibodies H.M.F.G.1. and H.M.F.G.2. in breast cancer. *Br. J. Cancer*, **51**, 179.

TUMOR METASTASIS: VASCULAR INVASION

Bettelheim, R. *et al.* (1984) Prognostic significance of peritumoral vascular invasion in breast cancer. *Br. J. Cancer*, **50**, 771.

Gilchrist, J.W. *et al.* (1982) Interobserver variation in the identification of breast carcinoma in intramammary lymphatics. *Hum. Pathol.*, **13**, 170.

Lee, A.K.C. *et al.* (1986) Lymphatic and blood vessel invasion in breast carcinoma. *Hum. Pathol.*, **17**, 984.

Nime, F.A. *et al.* (1977) Prognostic significance of tumor emboli in intramammary lymphatics in patients with mammary carcinoma. *Am. J. Surg. Pathol.*, **1**, 25.

TUMOR METASTASIS: STRIATED MUSCLE INVASION

Lasser, A. *et al.* (1982) Intraskeletal myofiber metastasis of breast carcinoma. *Hum. Pathol.*, **13**, 1045.

Sarma, D.P. *et al.* (1985) Intramyofiber metastasis in skeletal muscle. *J. Surg. Oncol.*, **30**, 103.

INTRADUCTAL STRUCTURE

Lagios, M.D. *et al.* (1982) Duct carcinoma in situ. Relationship of extent of non invasive disease to the frequency of occult invasion, multicentricity, lymph node metastases. *Cancer*, **50**, 1309.

Silverberg, S.G. *et al.* (1973) Assessment of significance of proportions in intraductal and infiltrating tumor growth in ductal carcinoma of the breast. *Cancer*, **32**, 830.

INVASIVE LOBULAR CARCINOMA

Al-Hariri, J.A. (1980) Primary signet-ring cell carcinoma of the breast. *Virchows Arch.* (Pathol. Anat.), **388**, 105.

Allenby, P.A. *et al.* (1986) Histiocytic appearance of metastatic lobular breast carcinoma. *Arch. Pathol. Lab. Med.*, **110**, 759.

Eusebi, V. *et al.* (1977) Morpho-functional differentiation in lobular carcinoma of the breast. *Histopathology*, **1**, 301.

Eusebi, V. *et al.* (1984) Apocrine differentiation in lobular carcinoma of the breast. *Hum. Pathol.*, **15**, 134.

Fisher, E.R. *et al.* (1985) Intraductal signet-ring carcinoma. *Cancer*, **55**, 2533.

Fisher, E.R. *et al.* (1977) Tubulolobular invasive breast cancer: a variant of lobular invasive cancer. *Hum. Pathol.*, **8**, 679.

Gad, A. *et al.* (1975) Lobular carcinoma of the breast: a special variant of mucin-secreting carcinoma. *J. Clin. Pathol.*, **28**, 711.

Harris, M. *et al.* (1984) A comparison of the metastatic pattern of infiltrating lobular carcinoma and infiltrating duct carcinoma of the breast. *Br. J. Cancer*, **50**, 23.

Harris, M. *et al.* (1978) Primary signet-ring cell carcinoma of the breast. *Histopathology*, **2**, 171.

Hood, C.I. *et al.* (1973) Metastatic mammary carcinoma in the eyelid with histiocytoid appearance. *Cancer*, **31**, 793.

Hull, M.T. *et al.* (1980) Signet-ring cell carcinoma of the breast. *Am. J. Clin. Pathol.*, **73**, 31.

Martinez, V. *et al.* (1979) Invasive lobular carcinoma of the breast: incidence and variants. *Histopathology*, **3**, 467.

Merino, M.J. *et al.* (1981) Signet-ring carcinoma of the female breast. *Cancer*, **48**, 1830.

Nesland, J.M. *et al.* (1985) Ultrastructural and immunohistochemical features of lobular carcinoma of the breast. *J. Pathol.*, **145**, 39.

Shousha, S. *et al.* (1986) Alveolar variant of invasive lobular carcinoma of the breast. *Am. J. Clin. Pathol.*, **85**, 1.

MUCINOUS CARCINOMA

Capella, C. *et al.* (1980) Endocrine differentiation in mucoid carcinoma of the breast. *Histopathology*, **4**, 613

Clayton, F. (1986) Pure mucinous carcinomas of breast. *Hum. Pathol.*, **17**, 34.

Ferguson, D.J.P. *et al.* (1986) An ultrastructural study of mucoid carcinoma of the breast. *Histopathology*, **10**, 1219.

Norris, H.J. *et al.* (1965) Prognosis of mucinous carcinoma of the breast. *Cancer*, **18**, 879.

Rosen, P.P. *et al.* (1980) Colloid carcinoma of the breast: analysis of 64 patients with long-term follow-up. *Am. J. Clin. Pathol.*, **73**, 304.

MEDULLARY CARCINOMA

Flores, L. *et al.* (1974) Host tumor relationships in medullary carcinoma of the breast. *Surg. Gynecol. Obstet.*, **139**, 683.

Harris, M. *et al.* (1986) The ultrastructure of medullary, atypical medullary and non-medullary carcinomas of the breast. *Histopathology*, **10**, 405.

Ridolfi, R.L. *et al.* (1977) Medullary carcinoma of the breast. *Cancer*, **40**, 1365.

PAPILLARY CARCINOMA

Fisher, E.R. *et al.* (1980) Pathologic findings from the National Surgical Adjuvant. Breast Project (Protocol n° 4). IV – invasive papillary cancer. *Am. J. Clin. Pathol.*, **73**, 313.

TUBULAR CARCINOMA

Carstens, P.H.B. *et al.* (1985) Tubular carcinoma of the breast. A long-term follow-up. *Histopathology*, **9**, 271.

Cooper, H.S. *et al.* (1978) Tubular carcinoma of the breast. *Cancer*, **42**, 2334.

Fisher, E.R. *et al.* (1983) Scar cancers: pathologic findings from the National Surgical Adjuvant Breast Project (Protocol 4). *Breast Cancer Res. Treat.*, **3**, 39.

Lagios, M.D. *et al.* (1980) Tubular carcinoma of the breast. *Am. J. Clin. Pathol.*, **73**, 25.

Van Bogaert, L.J. (1982) Clinicopathologic hallmarks of mammary tubular carcinoma. *Hum. Pathol.*, **13**, 558.

ADENOID CYSTIC CARCINOMA

Caselitz, J. *et al.* (1984) Coexpression of keratin and vimentin filaments in adenoid cystic carcinomas of salivary glands. *Virchows Arch. (Pathol. Anat.)*, **403**, 337.

Cavanzo, F.J. *et al.* (1969) Adenoid cystic carcinoma of the breast. *Cancer*, **24**, 740.

Chaudhry, A.P. *et al.* (1986) Histogenesis of adenoid cystic carcinoma of the salivary glands. *Cancer*, **58**, 72.

Peters, G.N. *et al.* (1982) Adenoid cystic carcinoma of the breast. *Cancer*, **52**, 680.

Wells, C.A. *et al.* (1986) Adenoid cystic carcinoma of the breast: a case with axillary lymph node metastasis. *Histopathology*, **10**, 415.

Zaloudek, C. *et al.* (1984) Adenoid cystic carcinoma of the breast. *Am. J. Clin. Pathol.*, **81**, 297.

APOCRINE CARCINOMA

Eusebi, V. *et al.* (1986) Apocrine carcinoma of the breast. *Am. J. Pathol.*, **123**, 532.

Mazoujian, G. *et al.* (1983) Immunohistochemistry of a gross cyst disease fluid protein of the breast (GCDFP-15). *Am. J. Pathol.*, **110**, 105.

METAPLASTIC CARCINOMA

Battifora, H. (1976) Spindle cell carcinoma. *Cancer*, **37**, 2275.

Bauer, T.W. *et al.* (1984) Spindle cell carcinoma of the breast. *Hum. Pathol.*, **15**, 147.

Berg,. J.W. *et al.* (1962) Stromal sarcomas of the breast. *Cancer*, **15**, 418.

Bogomoletz, W. (1982) Pure squamous cell carcinoma of the breast. *Arch. Pathol. Lab. Med.*, **106**, 57.

Eggers, J.W. *et al.* (1984) Squamous cell carcinoma of the breast. *Hum. Pathol.*, **15**, 526.

Gersell, D.J. (1981) Spindle cell carcinoma of the breast. *Hum. Pathol.*, **12**, 550.

Huvos, A.G. *et al.* (1973) Metaplastic breast carcinoma. *N.Y. State J. Med.*, **73**, 1078.

Kahn, L.B. *et al.* (1978) Carcinoma of the breast with metaplasia to chondrosarcoma. *Histopathology*, **2**, 93.

Kaufman, M.W. *et al.* (1984) Carcinoma of the breast with pseudosarcomatous metaplasia. *Cancer*, **53**, 1908.

Koui, J. *et al.* (1981) High-grade mucoepidermoid carcinoma of the breast. *Arch. Pathol. Lab. Med.*, **105**, 612.

Llombart-Bosch, A. *et al.* (1975) Malignant mixed osteogenic tumours of the breast. *Virchows Arch. (Pathol. Anat.)*, **366**, 1.

Patchefsky, A.S. *et al.* (1979) Low-grade mucoepidermoid carcinoma of the breast. *Arch. Pathol. Lab. Med.*, **103**, 196.

Rosen, P.P. *et al.* (1987) Low-grade adenosquamous carcinoma. *Am. J. Surg. Pathol.*, **11**, 351.

Toikhanen, S. (1981) Primary squamous cell carcinoma of the breast. *Cancer*, **48**, 1629.

Vera-Sempere, F.J. *et al.* (1985) Squamous carcinoma of the breast: pure and metaplastic variants. *Breast Diseases Senologia*, **1**, 81.

Woodard, B.H. *et al.* (1980) Adenosquamous differentiation in mammary carcinoma. *Arch. Pathol. Lab. Med.*, **104**, 130.

Zarbo, R.J. *et al.* (1986) Spindle cell carcinoma of the upper aerodigestive tract mucosa. *Am. J. Surg. Pathol.*, **10**, 741.

OTHER INVASIVE CARCINOMAS

Breast carcinoma with osteoclast-like giant cells

Agnantis, N.T. *et al.* (1979) Mammary carcinoma with osteoclast-like giant cells. *Am. J. Clin. Pathol.*, **72**, 383.

Holland, R. *et al.* (1984) Mammary carcinoma with osteoclast-like giant cells. *Cancer*, **53**, 1963.

McMahon, R.F. *et al.* (1986) Breast carcinoma with stromal multinucleated giant cells. *J. Pathol.*, **150**, 175.

Nielsen, B.B. *et al.* (1985) Carcinoma of the breast with stromal multinucleated giant cells. *Histopathology*, **9**, 183.

Tavassoli, F.A. *et al.* (1986) Breast carcinoma with osteoclast-like giant cells. *Arch. Pathol. Lab. Med.*, **110**, 636.

Secretory carcinoma

McDivitt, R.W. and Stewart, F.W. (1966) Breast carcinoma in children. *J.A.M.A.*, **195**, 388.

Tavassoli, F.A. and Norris, H.J. (1980) Secretory carcinoma of the breast. *Cancer*, **45**, 2404.

Glycogen-rich clear-cell carcinoma

Benisch, B. *et al.* (1983) Solid glycogen-rich clear cell carcinoma of the breast. *Am. J. Clin. Pathol.*, **79**, 243.

Fisher, E.R. *et al.* (1985) Glycogen-rich clear cell breast cancer: with comments concerning other clear cell variants. *Hum. Pathol.*, **16**, 1085.

Hull, M.T. *et al.* (1986) Glycogen-rich clear cell carcinomas of the breast. *Am. J. Surg. Pathol.*, **10** (8), 553.

A lipid-secreting carcinoma

Fisher, E.R. *et al.* (1977) Lipid in invasive cancer of the breast. *Am. J. Clin. Pathol.*, **68**, 558.

Ramos, C.V. *et al.* (1974) Lipid-rich carcinoma of the breast. *Cancer*, **33**, 812.

Van Bogaert, L.J. *et al.* (1977) Histologic variants of lipid-secreting carcinoma of the breast. *Virchows Arch.* (Pathol. Anat.), **375**, 345.

PAGET'S DISEASE OF THE NIPPLE

Kirkham, N. *et al.* (1985) Paget's disease of the nipple. *Cancer*, **55**, 1510.

Lagios, M.D. *et al.* (1984) Paget's disease of the nipple. *Cancer*, **54**, 545.

Ordonez, N.G. *et al.* (1987) Mammary and extramammary Paget's disease. *Cancer*, **59**, 1173.

COMBINATIONS OF HISTOLOGICAL TYPES
IN THE SAME TUMOUR MASS

Stenkvist, B. *et al.* (1985) Histopathological systems of breast cancer classification. *J. Clin. Pathol.*, **36**, 392.

Trojani, M. *et al.* (1984) Classification des cancers du sein. *Arch. Anat. Cytol. Pathol.*, **32**, 133.

Van Bogaert, L.J. *et al.* (1986) An analytic critique of existing classification systems for cancer of the breast. *Surg. Gynecol. Obstet.*, **142**, 513.

8
Miscellaneous malignant tumours

This chapter groups various malignant tumours of low incidence.

8.1 Angiosarcoma

They originate from mammary stromal elements and are similar to extramammary soft tissue sarcomas.

Angiosarcoma requires a particular mention because it is more frequent in the breast than at other sites in the body. With this exception, the most frequent sarcomas are liposarcoma, fibrosarcoma, malignant fibrohistiocytoma and undifferentiated high grade sarcoma.

The term 'stromal sarcoma' has been introduced by Berg (1962) to designate tumours arising from mammary gland connective tissue, excluding adjacent tissues (muscle, skin). This controversial term should be strictly applied to the very exceptional sarcomas arising from the specialized stroma of the breast (periductal or lobular stroma). Breast sarcomas must be distinguished from carcinosarcomas developed in cystosarcoma phyllodes and from metaplastic carcinomas.

8.2 Non-Hodgkin's malignant lymphoma with initial mammary localization.

8.3 Granulocytic sarcoma

8.4 Metastasis to the breast from a malignant tumour localized elsewhere.

8.1 ANGIOSARCOMA

Synonyms

Hemangioendothelioma, hemangioblastoma, hemangiosarcoma.

Definition

A rare and highly malignant tumour of vascular origin.

Clinical features

- Young women of childbearing age,
- Palpable tumour with poorly defined margins and rapid growth, sometimes bilateral.
- Very poor prognosis. Tumour size and degree of differentiation are probably the most important prognostic factors (early generalization and frequent localization in the gums).

Histological features

- Interanastomosing vascular channels
- Endothelial tufting and intraluminal papillary projections
- Solid, spindle-cell areas with mitoses, necrosis and hemorrhage

Immunohistochemical features

Factor VIII-related antigen: positive
Vimentin: positive
Epithelial markers: negative

Differential diagnosis: with a benign angioma, a carcinoma.

STEWART-TREVES SYNDROME

This usually corresponds to an angiosarcoma arising in the post-mastectomy lymphoedematous arms, but the histogenesis remains controversial: blood or lymphatic vascular origin, or metastasis from the original breast carcinoma or from a new primary tumour. This syndrome actually overlaps the two eventualities but immunohistochemical stainings should allow one to distinguish easily between them.

Two idioms have become classical with regard to vascular breast tumours:
1. **Any palpable vascular breast tumour is an a priori suspicion of malignancy (however some of them are apparently not malignant).**
2. **Angiosarcoma can have a benign histologic appearance: interanastomosing channels are a good criterion of malignancy in this case.**

541 HES ×10
Angiosarcoma: hemorrhagic tumour with multiple cystic blood-filled spaces.

542 HES ×64
Well-differentiated lesion = grade I.
Interanastomosing vascular spaces.

543 HES ×25
544 HES ×160
Moderately differentiated = grade II.
Predominance of endothelial tufting and papillary projections, with large hyperchromatic endothelial cells.

545 HES ×64
546 HES ×160
Poorly differentiated = grade III.
Predominance of solid areas with atypical spindle cells and mitoses.

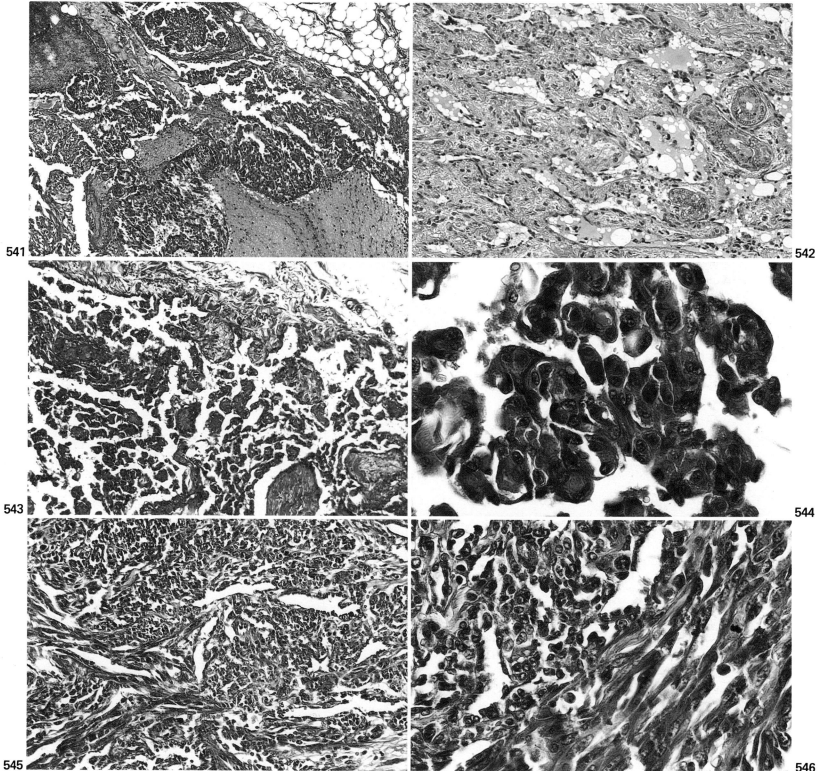

541

542

543

544

545

546

8.2 NON-HODGKIN'S MALIGNANT LYMPHOMA

The primary mammary site of lymphoma is very rare.

Clinical features

- mean age similar to that of breast carcinoma (57 years)
- voluminous and rapidly enlarging tumour accompanied by inflammatory signs.

Radiological features

- often benign aspect: sharply outlined nodule like a fibroadenoma or a phyllodes tumour,
- rarely nodule with ill-defined contour simulating a carcinoma.

Histological features

Histologic types are identical to those of other localizations.

Differential diagnosis

With a medullary or anaplastic carcinoma. Diagnosis is made easy by the positivity of leucocyte markers and the negativity of epithelial markers.

- **Contrast between the alarming clinical aspect and the mammographic benign aspect,**
- **Difficulty of diagnosis on frozen sections (mistaken for a carcinoma),**
- **Prognosis and treatment similar to those of lymphomas in other sites (depending on histologic type and extension).**

---

547 Mammography
Lobulated, well-circumscribed, radiopaque nodule (50mm) with benign appearance.

548 HES ×160
549 Giemsa ×160 } NHML (lymphoplasmocytoid type)

550 Cytok ×160
Negativity of tumour cells.

551 LCA ×160
Positivity of all cells.

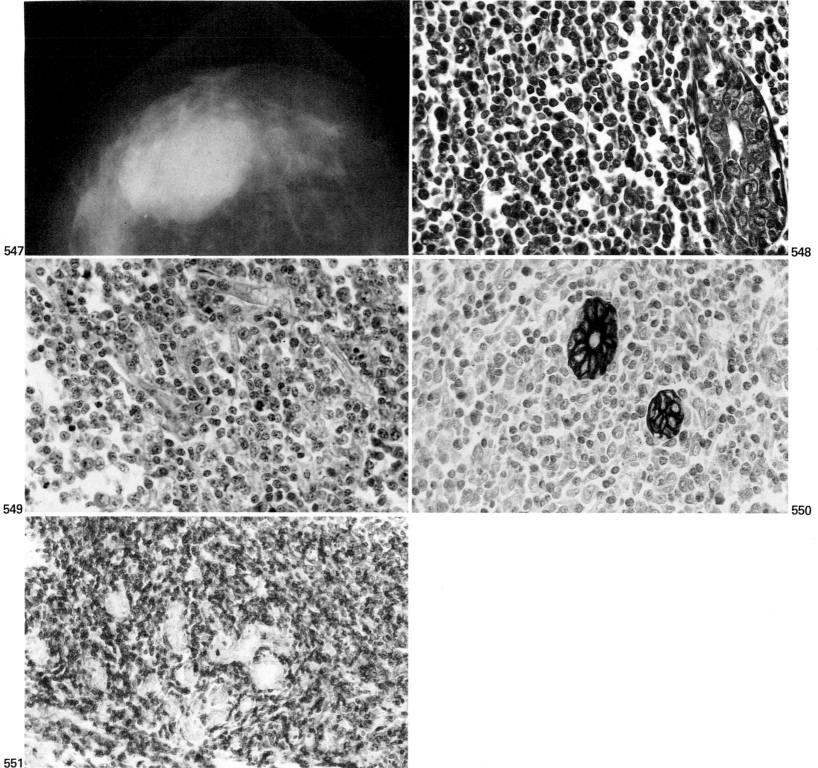

8.3 GRANULOCYTIC SARCOMA

Synonym

Chloroma, myeloblastoma.

Definition

Solid tumour composed of immature cells of the granulocytic series and corresponding to an extramedullary tumour variant of acute myeloid leukaemia (AML).

Clinical features

- More common in children and young adults.
- Site: subperiosteal bone (skull, orbit, ribs), organs (kidney, ovary, breast), lymph nodes.
- Always associated with a disseminated leukaemia: most often, granulocytic sarcoma and leukaemia occur simultaneously, but the sarcoma may precede the leukaemia of a few months or very rarely occur in the course of it.

Histological features

- Pseudolymphomatous appearance but as opposed to lymphoma, presence of eosinophilic myelocytes in the neoplasm.
- Reactivity in tissue sections for chloracetate esterase revealed by the Leder stain, for lysozyme and other granulocytic markers (CD15).

Differential diagnosis

With a lymphoma, helped by enzymatic and immunohistochemical staining techniques, sometimes by electron microscopy.

552 HES ×160
Pseudolymphomatous proliferation.

553 Giemsa ×400
Tumour cells with prominent nucleoli and large cytoplasms in which very small eosinophilic granules are visible.

554 MGG ×400
Tissue imprints:
Numerous azurophilic granules in tumour cells, characteristic of myeloid cells.

8.4 METASTASIS TO THE BREAST FROM A MALIGNANT TUMOUR LOCALIZED ELSEWHERE

Tumours metastatic to the breast are rare. In adults, the most frequent origin is malignant melanoma and carcinoids; in children, round-cell tumours (embryonal rhabdomyosarcoma, Ewing's sarcoma, neuroblastoma).

An intramammary metastasis is difficult to diagnose when it is the first manifestation of an occult cancer or the solitary secondary localization of a known cancer. It may be solitary for a long time and mistaken for a primary breast cancer.

555 Mammography
Large nodule (65mm) with high density and sharply outlined contour, adherent to the skin.

556 HES ×160
Malignant melanocytic cells with melanin deposit.

557 S100 protein
Cytoplasmic positivity of all tumour cells.

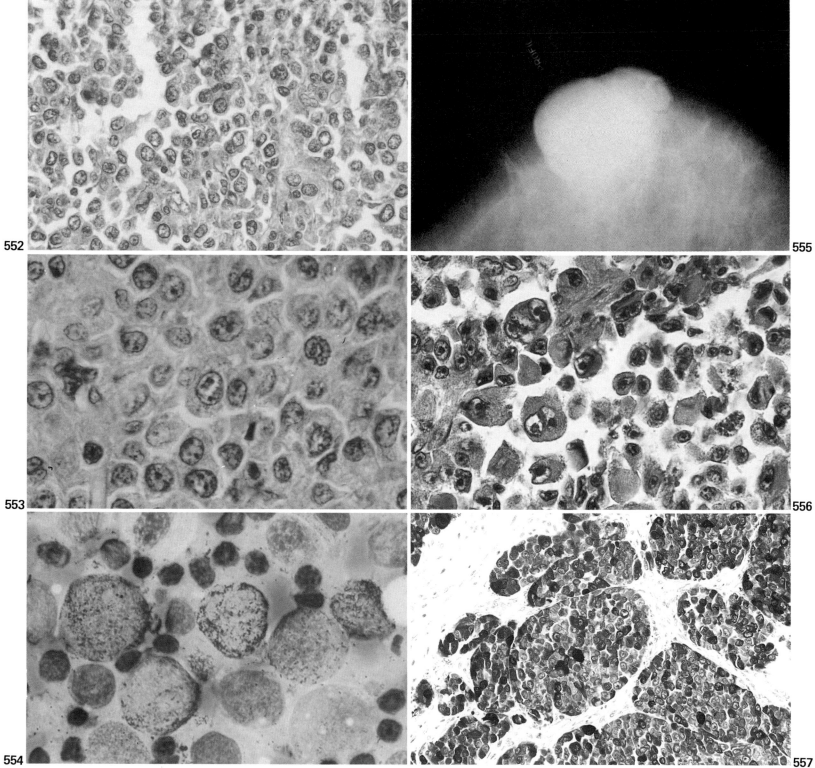

552

555

553

556

554

557

References
Chap. 8 – Miscellaneous Malignant Tumours

Sarcoma

Austin, R.M. *et al.* (1986) Liposarcoma of the breast. *Hum. Pathol.*, **17**, 906.

Berg, J.W. *et al.* (1962) Stromal sarcomas of the breast. *Cancer*, **15**, 418.

Callery, C.D. *et al.* (1985) Sarcoma of the breast. *Ann. Surg.*, **201**, 527.

Mufarrij, A.A. *et al.* (1987) Breast sarcoma with giant cells and osteoid. *Am. J. Surg. Parthol.*, **11**, 225.

Norris, H.J. and Taylor, H.B. (1968) Sarcomas and related mesenchymal tumors of the breast. *Cancer*, **22**, 22.

Angiosarcoma – Stewart-Treves Syndrome

Chen, K.T.K. *et al.* (1980) Angiosarcoma of the breast. *Cancer*, **46**, 368.

Donnell, R.M. *et al.* (1981) Angiosarcoma and other vascular tumors of the breast. *Am. J. Surg. Pathol.*, **5**, 629.

Govoni, E. *et al.* (1981) Post-mastectomy angiosarcoma: ultrastructural study of a case. *Tumori*, **67**, 79.

Hunter, T.B. *et al.* (1985) Angiosarcoma of the breast. *Cancer*, **56**, 2099.

Merino, M.J. *et al.* (1983) Angiosarcoma of the breast. *Am. J. Surg. Pathol.*, **7**, 53.

Schafler, K. *et al.* (1979) Post-mastectomy lymphangiosarcoma. *Histopathology*, **3**, 131.

Sordillo, P.P. *et al.* (1981) Lymphangiosarcoma. *Cancer*, **48**, 1674.

Non-Hodgkin's malignant lymphoma – Granulocyte sarcoma

André, J.M. *et al.* (1983) Lymphomes malins et autres hématosarcomes à localisation mammaire initiale. *Bull. Cancer* (Paris), **70**, 401.

Brustein, S. *et al.* (1987) Malignant lymphoma of the breast. *Ann. Surg.*, **205**, 144.

Gartenhaus, W.S. *et al.* (1985) Granulocytic sarcoma of the breast. *Med. Pediatr. Oncol.*, **13**, 22.

Nieman, R.S. *et al.* (1981) Granulocytic sarcoma: a clinicopathologic study of 61 biopsied cases. *Cancer*, **48**, 1426.

Sears, H.F. *et al.* (1976) Granulocytic sarcoma. *Cancer*, **37**, 1808.

Telesinghe, P.U. *et al.* (1985) Primary lymphoma of the breast. *Histopathology*, **9**, 297.

Wiernik, P. *et al.* (1970) Granulocytic sarcoma. *Blood*, **35**, 361.

Intramammary metastasis

Hadju, S.I. *et al.* (1972) Cancers metastatic to the breast. *Cancer*, **29**, 1691.

Howarth, C.B. *et al.* (1980) Breast metastases in children with rhabdomyosarcoma. *Cancer*, **46**, 2520.

Kashlan, R.B. *et al.* (1982) Carcinoid and other tumours metastatic to the breast. *J. Surg. Oncol.*, **20**, 25.

Pressman, P.L. (1973) Malignant melanoma and the breast. *Cancer*, **21**, 784.

9
Axillary lymph node

9.1 LYMPH NODE METASTASIS

Axillary lymph nodes are the first and main stage of the lymphatic routes of breast cancer. The number of metastatic lymph nodes is an important factor in predicting prognosis and guiding treatment.

Lymph node invasion may be partial or total, with or without capsular rupture. It may also be very small as micrometastases. The detection of micro-metastases can be improved by serial sections and immunohistochemical staining.

> Note: in lymph node metastases of invasive lobular carcinoma, tumour cells are not readily visible by routine staining and are often mistaken for histiocytes.

IDC METASTASIS

558 HES ×10
Total invasion with fibrous stromal reaction.

559 HES ×10
Subcapsular metastasis with a pseudopapillary lymphatic invasion.

560 Cytok ×160
Small metastatic island in the subcapsular sinus.

ILC METASTASIS

561 HES ×64
Total invasion by single cells within a fibrous stroma.

562 HES ×25
Single cells intermingled with lymphocytes may give the appearance of a malignant lymphoma (often not recognized if only present in small numbers).

563 Cytok ×64
Strong positivity of the ILC cells disseminated throughout the lymphoid tissue. These cells had not been detected by conventional staining.

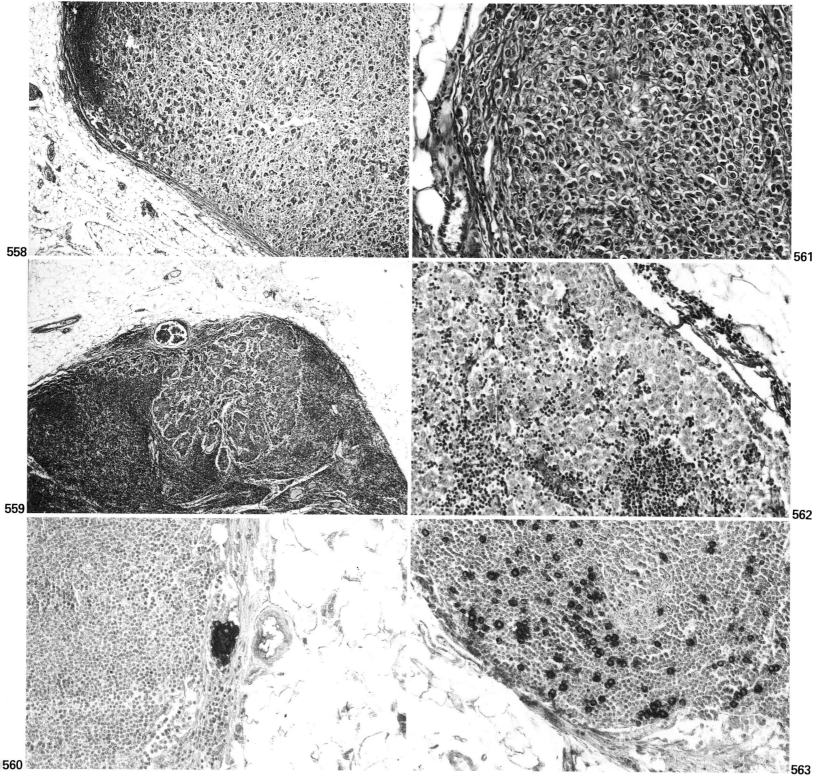

558

561

559

562

560

563

9.2 BENIGN INCLUSIONS IN AXILLARY LYMPH NODES

Benign mammary tissue may be found in axillary lymph nodes and must be distinguished from metastatic carcinoma, but these ectopic structures lack malignant cytological features and are heterogeneous with glandular structures, apocrine cysts and squamous cysts. Sometimes the glands have two cell layers or apical snouts.

564 HES ×25
565 HES ×64
566 HES ×64
Benign mammary tissue; glands with apocrine snouts, epitheliosis and an apocrine cyst.

Naevus cells in axillary lymph nodes are found in the capsule and sometimes in the fibrous trabeculae within the node, exceptionally within the parenchyma. They must not be mistaken for metastatic carcinoma. The diagnosis is helped by S100 protein reactivity and epithelial antigen negativity.

567 HES ×64
568 S100 protein ×5
569 S100 protein ×64
Naevus cells in capsule and trabeculae, strongly reactive with S100 protein staining.

References
Chap. 9 – Axillary Lymph Nodes

I. LYMPH NODE METASTASIS

Contesso, G. *et al.* (1975) L'envahissement ganglionnaire locorégional des cancers du sein. *Bull. Cancer*, **62**, 359.

Hartveit, D. *et al.* (1982) Routine histological investigation of the axillary nodes in breast cancer. *Clin. Oncol.*, **8**, 121.

Rosen, P.P. *et al.* (1983) Discontinuous or 'skip' metastases in breast carcinoma. *Ann. Surg.*, **197**, 276.

Trojani, M. *et al.* (1987) Micrometastases to axillary lymph nodes from carcinoma of breast. Detection by immunohistochemistry and prognostic significance. *Br. J. Cancer*, **55**, 303.

II. BENIGN INCLUSIONS IN AXILLARY LYMPH NODES

Bertrand, G. *et al.* (1980) Présence de cellules naeviques dans les ganglions lymphatiques. *Arch. Anat. Cytol. Pathol.*, **28**, 58.

Turner, D.R. *et al.* (1980) Breast tissue inclusions in axillary lymph nodes. *Histopathology*, **4**, 631.

Yazdi, H.M. (1985) Nevus cells aggregates associated with lymph nodes. *Arch. Pathol. Lab. Med.*, **109**, 1044.

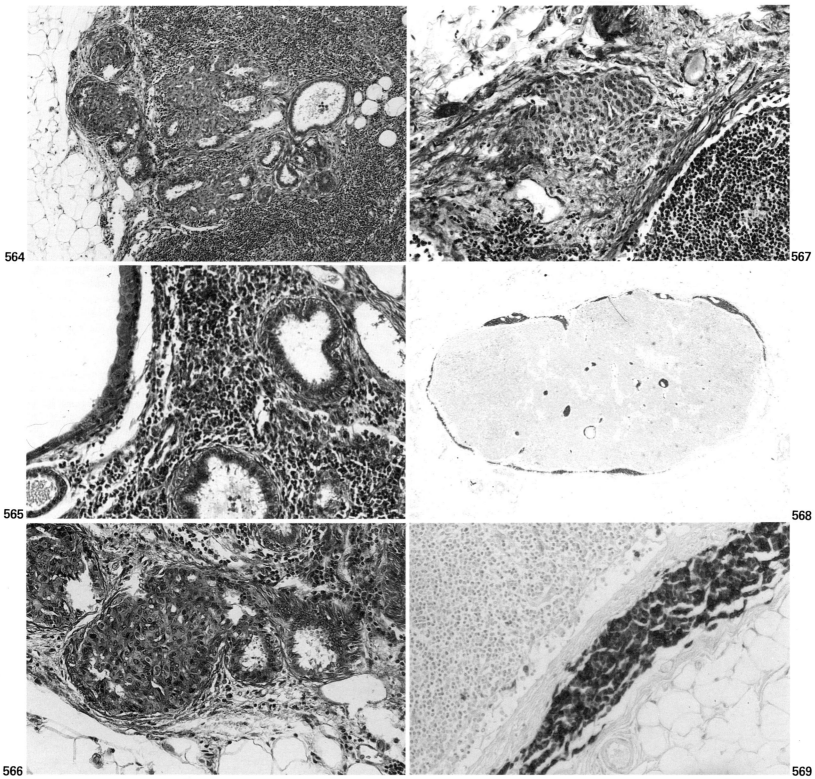

Index

Aubin Imprimeur Ligugé-Poitiers
Achevé d'imprimer en novembre 1990
Dépôt légal, novembre 1990 / Nᵒ d'impression P 36444
Printed in France